第1回全世界フルコンタクト空手道選手権大会

WFKO SELECTION TOURNAMENT

EUROPEAN FULLCONTACT KARATE CUP

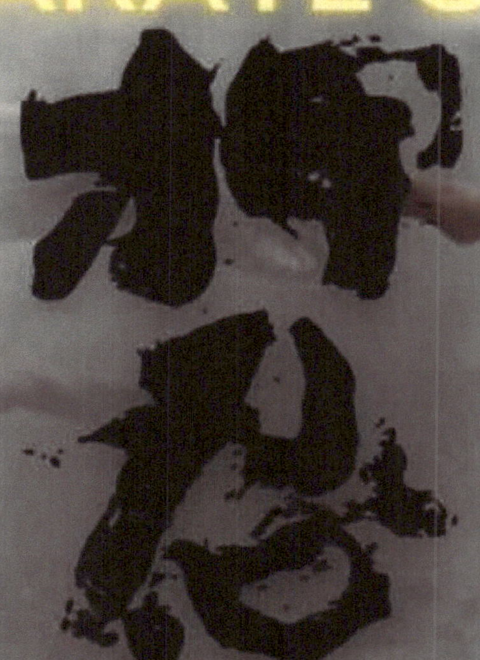

23 / 24 NOVEMBER 2024

ARENA HAL ANTWERP

Adults Men -60, -70, -80, -90, +90
Adults Women -50, -54, -59, -65, +65

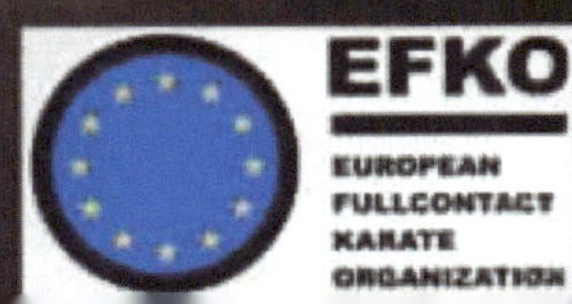

www.efko.info

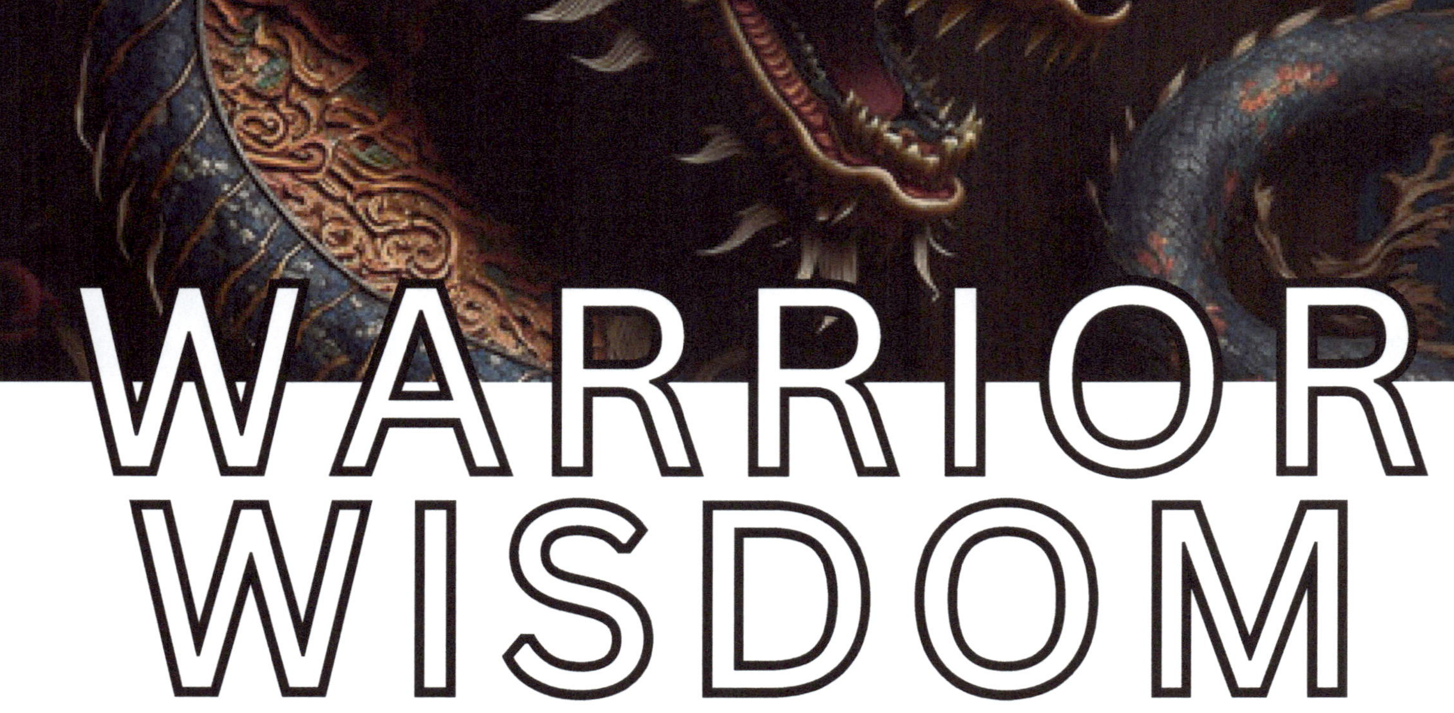

WARRIOR WISDOM

True Self-Defense Leaves Nothing Out!

Bohdi Sanders, Ph.D.

When most people hear the term "self-defense," it brings up visions of being physically attacked on the street or in a bar, or maybe a home invasion. This is especially true of martial artists. Hardcore martial artists train for self-defense, not as a hobby or as a sport. We practice hard, visualizing the poor thug who was crazy enough to attack us and seeing ourselves totally dismantling our attacker.

Likewise, many martial artists have a false idea about what forms and katas are all about. They are essentially self-defense practice as well, but only if you visualize yourself being attacked as you perform your kata. This is the true bunkai, the practical application, of all katas and forms. They are practice against multiple attackers.

Many martial artists see their forms as simply memorizing a sequence of specific blocks, kicks, and punches, but they are missing out on the true essence of their forms. If they simply see their forms as a specific sequence of stances, blocks, kicks, and punches that they must memorize to advance to a higher belt rank, they don't truly understand their art.

Although many dojos have lost the true meaning of martial arts, that doesn't change the fact that martial arts actually mean the art of war. They were never meant to be a cool type of exercise or a sport.

Furthermore, the art of war and complete self-defense are not entirely the same thing. The art of war encompasses the physical aspects and strategies of the martial arts.

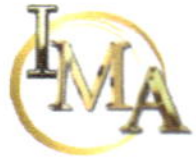

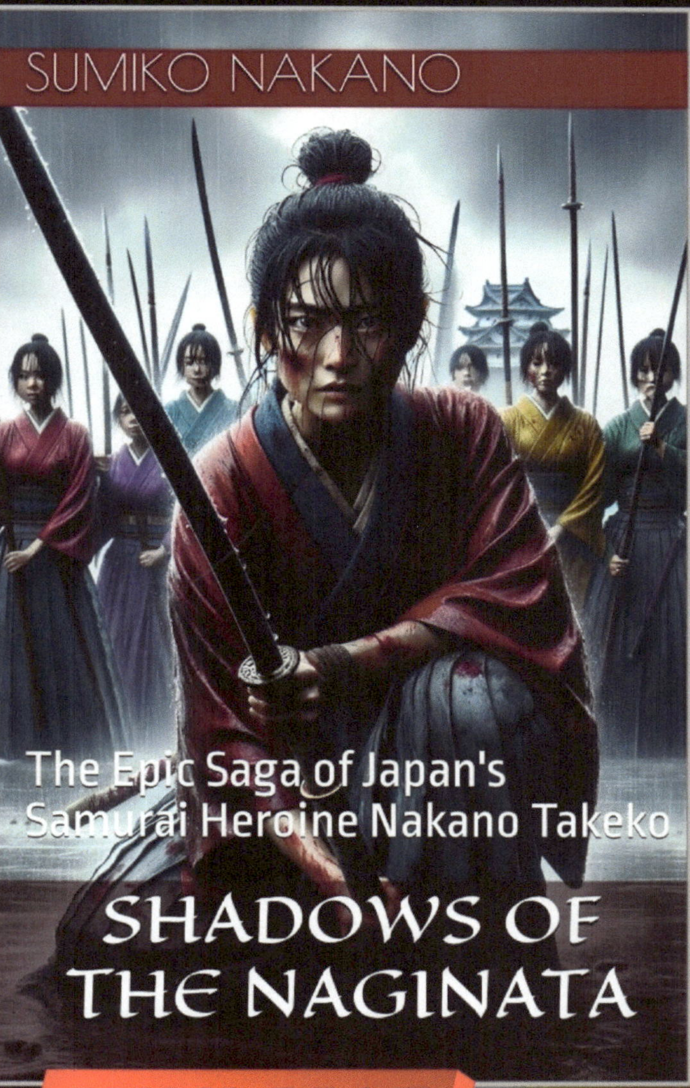

SUMIKO NAKANO
The Epic Saga of Japan's
Samurai Heroine Nakano Takeko
SHADOWS OF
THE NAGINATA

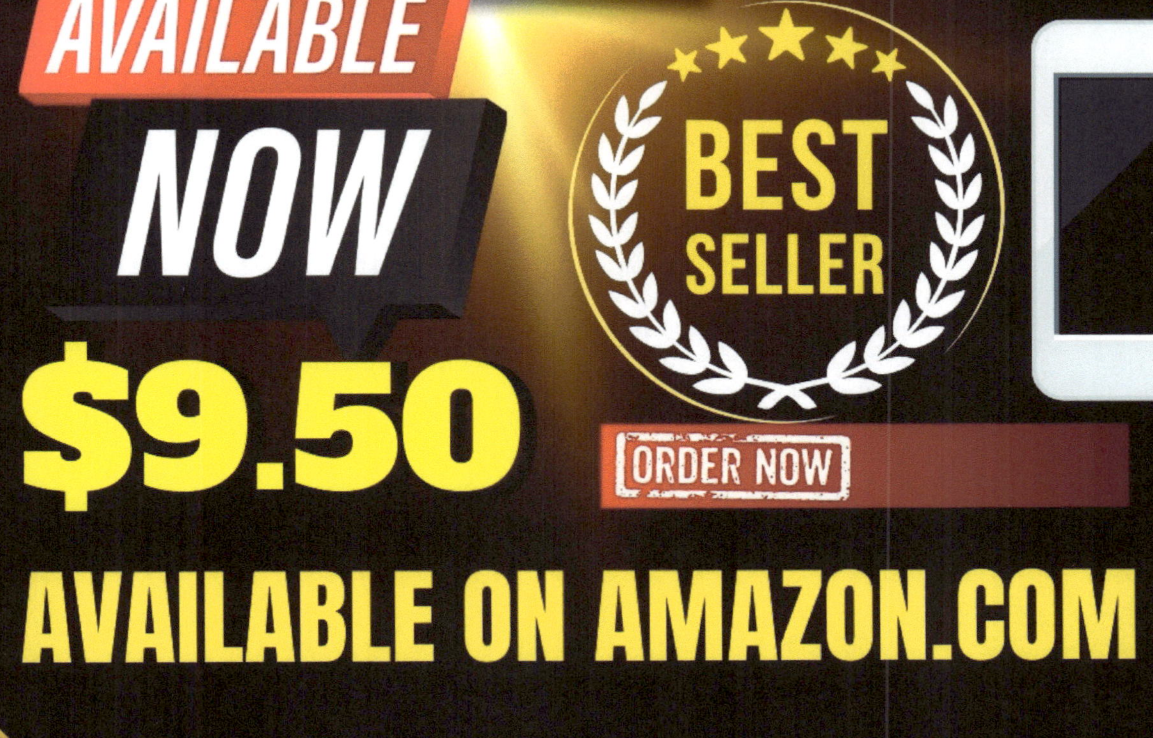

AVAILABLE
NOW
BEST
SELLER
ORDER NOW
$9.50
AVAILABLE ON AMAZON.COM

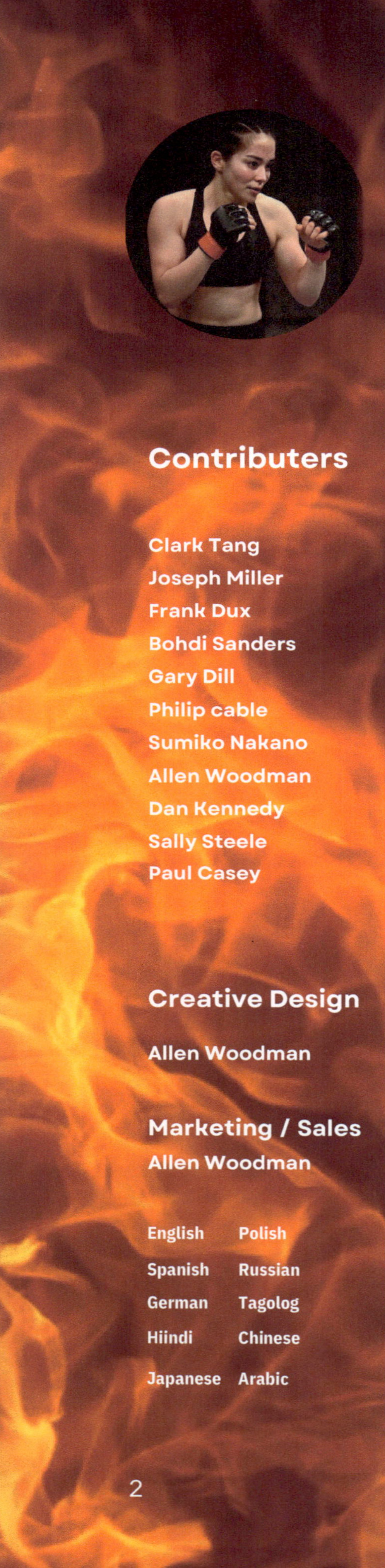

ABOUT THE COVER

On the cover of this month's issue of
INTERNATIONAL MARTIAL ARTS MAGAZINE
Sumiko Nakano

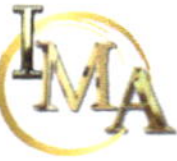

TABLE OF
Contents
INTERNATIONAL MARTIAL ARTS MAGAZINE

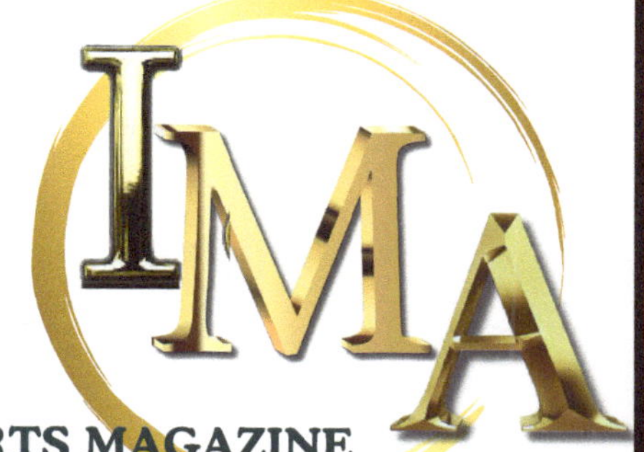

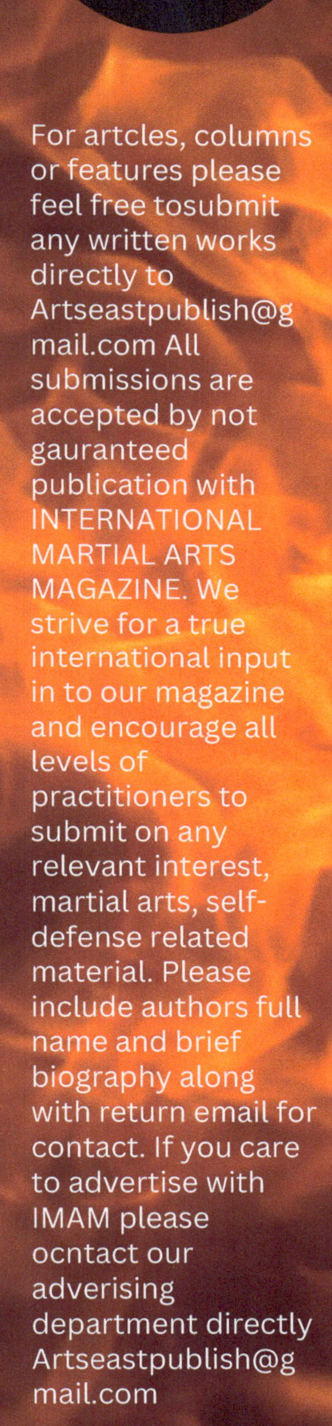

For artcles, columns or features please feel free tosubmit any written works directly to Artseastpublish@gmail.com All submissions are accepted by not gauranteed publication with INTERNATIONAL MARTIAL ARTS MAGAZINE. We strive for a true international input in to our magazine and encourage all levels of practitioners to submit on any relevant interest, martial arts, self-defense related material. Please include authors full name and brief biography along with return email for contact. If you care to advertise with IMAM please ocntact our adverising department directly Artseastpublish@gmail.com

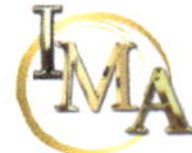

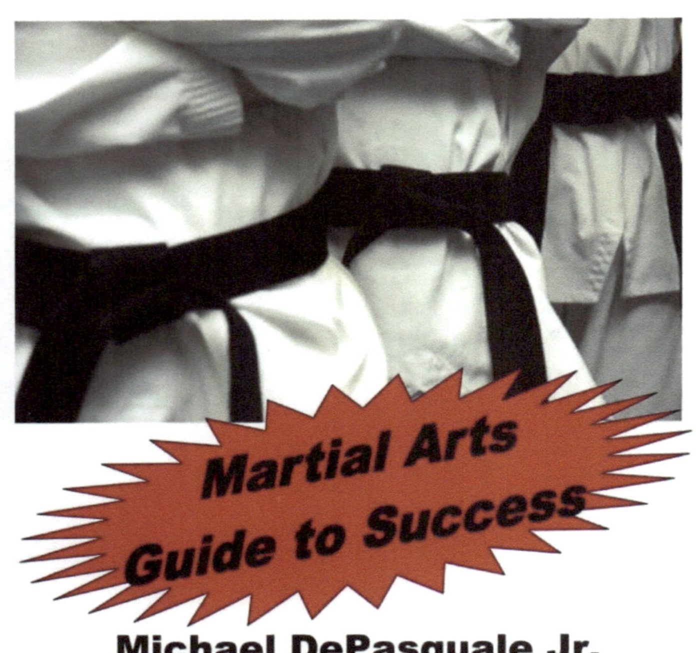

MARTIAL ARTS GUIDE TO SUCCESS

$19.95

Soke Michael DePasquale Jr. & Shihan Allen Woodman bring you a true perspective and practical business sense to open, run and effectively manage a martial arts school.

With over 80 years combined knowledge in owning, managing and instructing martial arts schools nationwide.

- ✓ Lease negotiations
- ✓ Daily management solutions
- ✓ How to get free advertisement for your school.
- ✓ Learn how to attract students and keep them.
- ✓ Techniques to help cover overhead cost
- ✓ Earning more money, doing the same things you do now.

The information you need today to take your school into the next decade and become financially strong.

ORDER NOW

328 pages
Language-English
Publication date
January 1, 2012
Dimensions
8.5 x 0.69 x 11

AVAILABLE ON AMAZON.COM

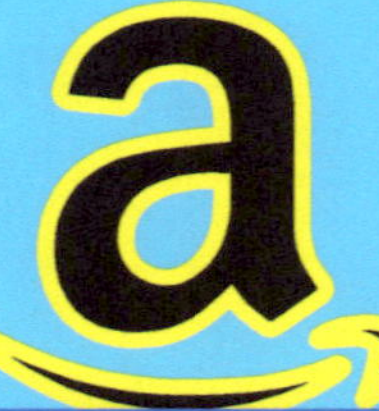

And, although the art of war parallels and overlaps with the art of self-defense, they are not completely the same thing. For example, in today's world, there are many ways that someone can harm you or your family that have nothing to do with the physical side of self-defense. Many martial artists who are in the public eye or who have rivals in their local area are familiar with the underhanded tactics used by their unscrupulous rivals.

Many unscrupulous people will attack your reputation and your name by using underhanded tactics on the internet or social media to destroy your reputation. This also goes on in various workplaces where a colleague may undermine you to cost you a promotion, or even cost you your job. These things are much more common than you may think.

I could give you example after example of martial artists who have been attacked in this cowardly way. You may think that this is just the actions of a coward, and you would be right. But whether you are dealing with a physical attack or a cowardly online attack, you still need to know how to protect yourself.

While an online attack or the underhanded strategy of a colleague may not harm you physically, they can do a lot of damage to you and your family. You need to learn how to defend yourself in those situations as well.

In addition, every martial artist must understand the laws and political climate in their country. Even if you are able to physically defend yourself against a physical attack, you still must do so in the right way to avoid being arrested and prosecuted by some distorted justice system.

Here in the United States, there are several examples of upstanding warriors and ex-military guys who have stepped in to protect innocent people who are being harassed, threatened, or attacked, only to be arrested for doing the right thing by a politicized justice system.

This is a reality that modern warriors must deal with and understand how to protect themselves from.

We live in times where doing the right thing can get you arrested and cost you thousands of dollars, while criminals and thugs can assault people, rob people, and destroy property without any worries of being arrested or prosecuted.

All of these are included under the category of self-defense. But most martial arts classes do not touch on these subjects, and if they do, it is simply a short warning like, "You must stop attacking when you have your attacker controlled or disabled, or you could be arrested."

The great teachers and sages all warned against these other types of attacks. Gichin Funakoshi stated, "In battle, do not think that you have to win. Think rather that you do not have to lose." You don't have to fight against every possible danger; just prepare yourself so well that you don't lose, and that it cannot hurt you.

Sun Tzu put it perfectly when he wrote, "The art of war teaches us to rely not on the likelihood of the enemy's not coming, but on our own readiness to receive him; not on the chance of his not attacking, but rather on the fact that we have made our position unassailable."

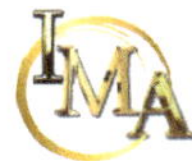

The truth of the matter is that we are far more likely to be targeted in these other ways than we are to be physically attacked on the streets.

Martial artists, who keep themselves in shape and carry themselves in a confident manner, are not the people that most criminals and predators on the street want to target. Predators are experts at sizing up their marks; the last thing they want to do is to attack someone who could beat the hell out of them.

On the other hand, any gutless coward can attack you online or take steps to destroy your reputation. They can covertly do things to undermine you and that will cost you dearly. And our legal system has become so unpredictable and corrupt that you should do everything in your power to stay clear of it.

A simple mistake or even doing the right thing, but in a careless way, can destroy your family and your finances. As Master Funakoshi taught, "Calamity springs from carelessness."

The true martial artist should be clearheaded and aware of all of these aspects of self-defense, and more. This means you must do whatever it takes to ensure your safety and the safety of your family and those around you.

While you should definitely hone your martial arts skills against a physical attack, you should also be aware that there are more ways that criminals and predators can hurt you. You must understand how to defend yourself against all forms of danger, not just the physical ones.

Never think that because you can protect yourself physically, that you are safe from danger. Danger comes in many forms. Some of them, like a venomous snake, are completely camouflaged and can catch you unaware or unprepared. I wrote Defensive Living: The Other Side of Self-Defense, several years ago to address these other forms of personal attacks.

Take steps to ensure that you are as safe and secure as possible. If you are only prepared for a physical attack, you have a large hole in your defense. True self-defense leaves nothing out! Warrior up!

Bohdi Sanders

Bohdi Sanders has been a martial artist for over 40 years, and is the author of 17 books on martial arts and warrior philosophy. His books are available on: www.TheWisdomWarrior.com and on Amazon. Bohdi can be reached at: WarriorWisdom@comcast.net.

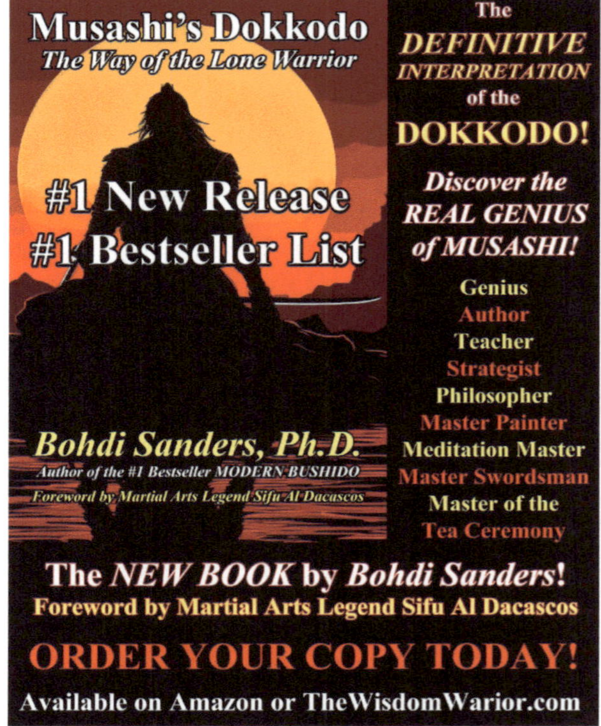

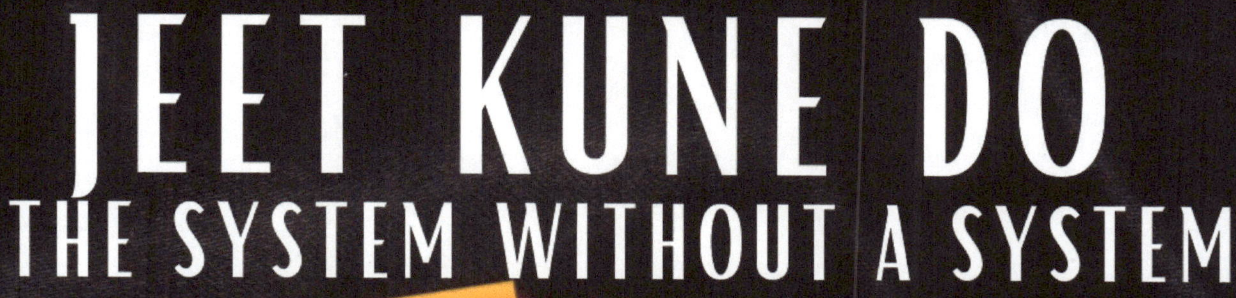

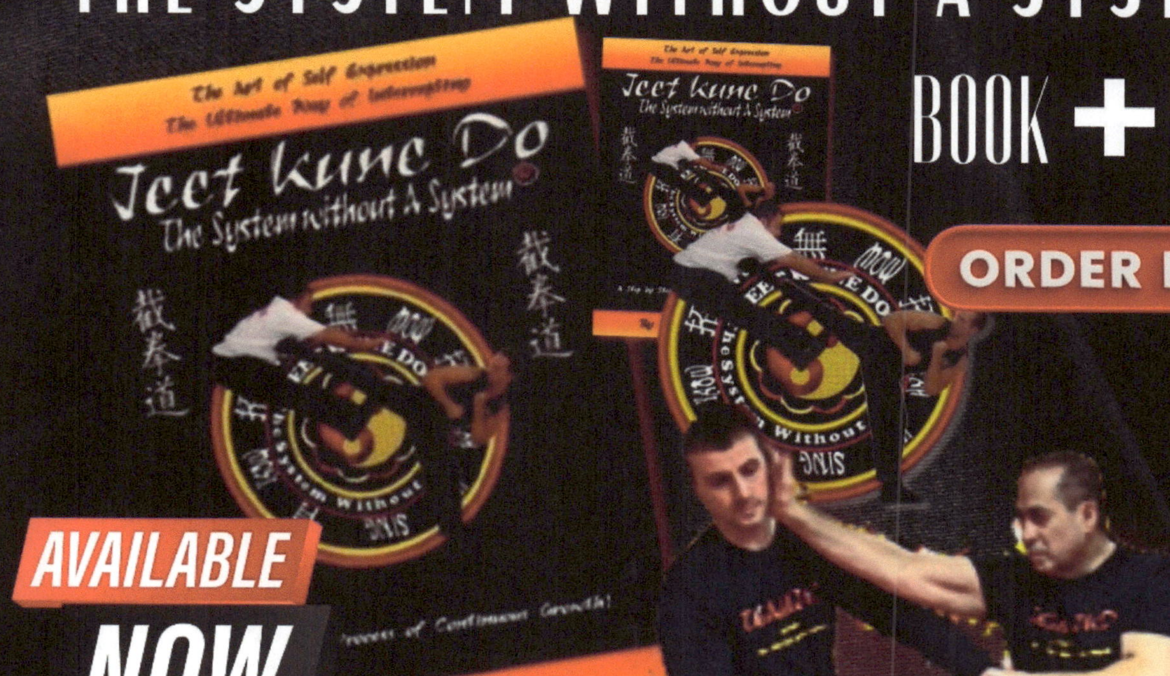

502 pages
Language English
Publication February 3, 2014
Dimensions 8.5 x 1.01 x 11.02
Jeet Kune Do A System Without a System is one of the best books ever written on the complete system that was pioneered by the late great Bruce Lee. George Hajnasr has put together the full course and understanding principles that are the make up of the complete system. Everything from Warm Up exercises to self defense techniques ranging from beginner to advanced. You will find it all in this one large manual of the Complete system of Jeet Kune DO A System Without a System.

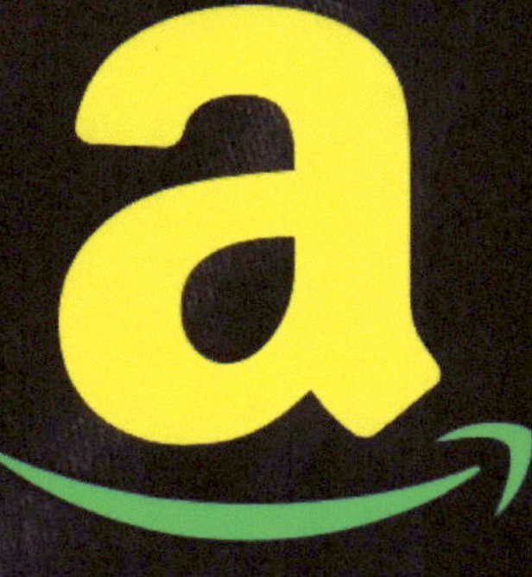

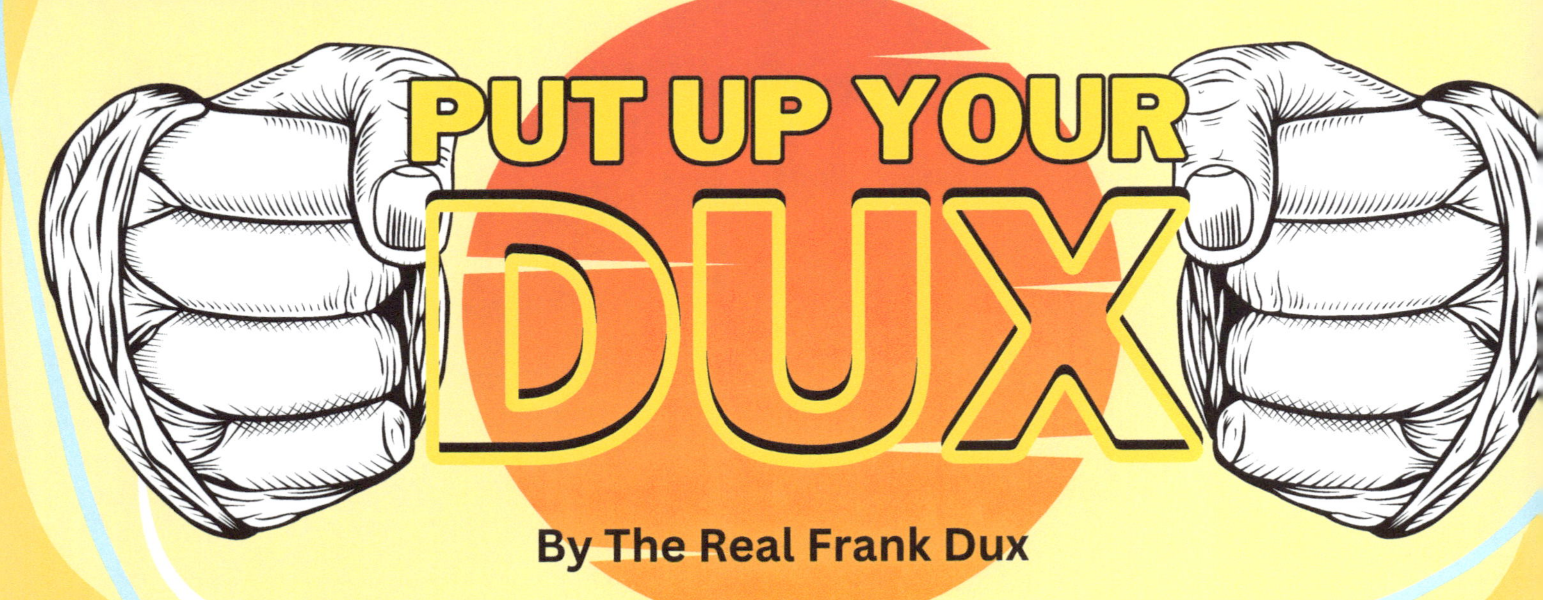

OWN THE INNER COWARD

Authentic admiration only comes to those that master the voice of cowardice, in them.

Reasonable fear is, good. It heightens awareness and prepares our body to fight or take flight. It can equally cause you to freeze up, resulting in serious bodily injury or death.

Being controlled by their inner coward is why most people end up filled with regret. They look back and then view their lives as an unfulfilled empty promise.

Fearlessness and ferocity are the signature traits of students of Dux Ryu. My training hall was in the heart of California's San Fernando Valley aka the legendary "Valley of Champions."

The Valley was home to a conglomeration of the greatest martial art icons at that time, in history.

Within walking distance of my humble 1400 sq ft. storefront business, was legendary PKA Kickboxing World Champion, Benny "The Jet" Urquidez. Who transformed a massive bowling alley into what was then a massive state of the art kickboxing gym called "The Jet Center."

Benny and I without trying shared students and even instructors because we were both stubbornly, uncompromising. In that, Benny and I taught martial arts the way it is always meant to be taught -- transformative.

No short cuts. No making everyone feel inclusive in handing out rank promotions and participation trophies. No fooling people into thinking inside 100 days with their first belt promotion they are a legit martial artist. When in 99 percent of the cases this attainment is not remotely, possible.

The legendary Mike Stone and Joe Lewis possibly being considered as exceptions to this rule.

However, their rough upbringings provided them with the spiritual strength inherent in a genuine martial artist.

The reason it takes years to be a genuine martial artist is because alive in each of us is that inner coward. Authentic martial arts instruction doesn't eliminate fear but provides the empirical experience and correct tools to cope with it.

Here are some tools when applied and used unconsciously will own your inner coward that defines your identity as an authentic martial artist.

1. Own your inner coward!

Acknowledging each one of our fears (like getting punched in the face) is the first step to controlling it and yourself.

It is painful and shameful to realize how fear driven and inauthentic we are or can become when we don't own our inner coward. That shows up when you make excuses for your piss-poor performance.

Don't be the guy who sucks at sparring, saying oh, my strike would blind and kill that opponent! That's like excusing away your chronically being not on-time for your MA class, lying to yourself "traffic is to blame" when bad planning or being easily distracted is the real reason. Something maybe you won't admit to, afraid of the teachers or classmate's reactions.

Giving into that inner coward makes us not trustworthy with ourselves. You can't build internal strength of character in the absence of confidence and self-esteem.

Without those attributes you end up trapped in a vicious circle of self-delusion, roleplaying the martial artist, Black Belt, etc.

Pressure-test yourself and your tools.

2. Spiritual Strength Training, always comes first!

Transcending our natural inclination for selfishness (which is another form of cowardice) is both a daily and a life-long obligation.

Give your spiritual training priority. A strong spirit prevents your inner coward from overtaking you when fear rises as a whisper of doubt—becomes what Buddhist monks refer to as: "The Chattering Monkeys in Your Head."

Meditation, visualization, prayer, comradery, strengthens and prepares our spirit for handling conflict.

Spiritual preparedness enhances our capability to "self-talk" that which enables us to adapt, remain organized in our thoughts and actions amid chaos, like violence.

If you fail to prepare to meet your spiritual battles you are not facing yourself. But hiding behind a rank or title (i.e. Sempai, Sensei, Sifu, Soke, etc.) to create a false sense of self-worth.

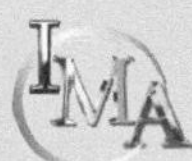

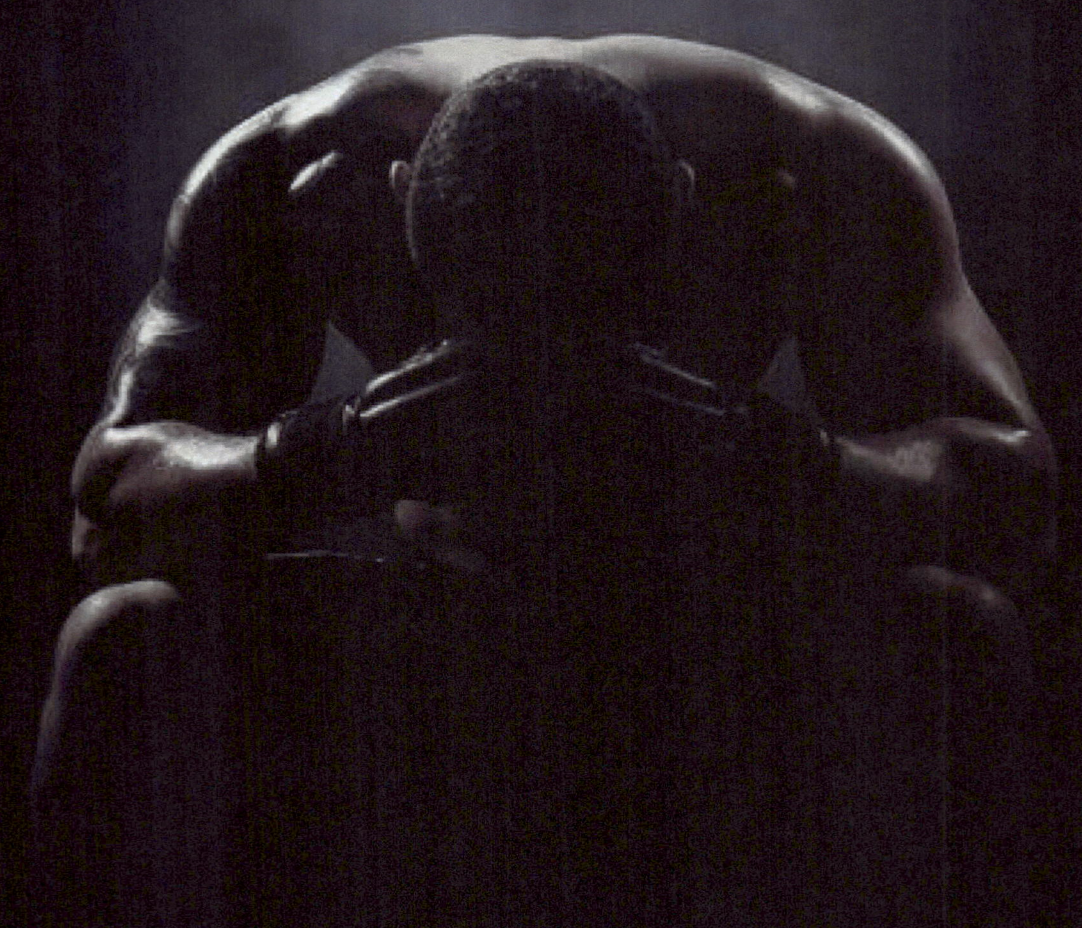

"Each of us must confront our own fears, must come face to face with them. How we handle our fears will determine where we go with the rest of our lives. To experience adventure or to be limited by the fear of it."

–Judy Blume

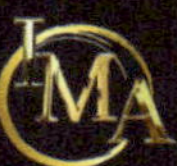

Uncompromising terms defines your identity. Uncompromising terms (i.e. you would never date any friends-ex) compromised by you will always cause you to feel lessened by the experience. Romantic break-ups are the best example of this reality.

The anger you experienced is proportionate to the compromises you made violating your own terms in or for that relationship.

3. Keep your word and actions aligned!

There is no gap between what you agree to and how you should perform. It is conniving cowardice that paints a favorable self-image, cause a person to say anything that sounds right, in the moment.

Being politically correct in an immoral situation is symptomatic of being owned by your fear. This shows up in changing your mind, frequently. Making excuses.

Trying to avoid commitment or excusing yourself away from previous promises, regularly.

Those are all indicators of someone running away from their true nature. A lack of strong character. Unwilling, to stand by their espoused convictions. That the coward in them, owns them.

Don't become that coward that will run away from the fight that can't be won but must be fought. "Remember the Alamo" and "Come and Take It" is the battle cry of the few and the brave.

4. Don't put yourself, first and foremost. Be capable of sacrifice!

Self-preservation at all costs is the domain of the coward.

The genuine martial artist accepts that battles fought are not just about them.

The "separated self" from the whole is a mindset that gives your self-preservation, priority. The kind to cause you to run away when a battle must be fought in the face of overwhelming odds.

Ask yourself are most of your actions aimed at creating something beneficial for yourself? Say hi, to your coward within.

5. Develop and maintain the offensive mindset, fearlessness!

An authentic martial artist takes educated risks. A good example is attempting to break a brick with a headbutt. This risks injury but so does headbutting a hard head. Living in denial of your fear by your avoiding fearful situations as in training to use a headbutt but never striking anything hard and forcefully with your forehead -- looking for comfort and chasing desire, you are living the cowardly life.

6. Don't "fake it to make it;" DO NOT live behind a mask!

Figuratively speaking, the coward wears several masks in projecting how they want to be perceived: successful; attractive; being cool – these are the favorites. Masks making someone appear intelligent and charming are, convenient.

It is now common sight that so called martial art teachers with no measurable accomplishments frequently pay for honor events where they engage in martial art style and rank certificate swapping.

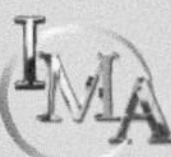

Getting their photo taken with most every celebrity attending to manipulate others perception of them. The signature of an authentic martial artist is their humility. This is because to be resilient when you experience failure you must be comfortable in your own skin.

Don't be the waiter who at parties introduce themselves as being a Hollywood producer, director, screenwriter, etc. when you have no professional work credits.

Be aware of your putting on airs. What are your masks? Are you committed to an unconditional discarding of wearing masks -- tossing aside manipulated perceptions, one after the other? If that is not to be the case, then arguably you are looking through the lens of a coward.

7. Don't hesitate when asked to help!

A genuine martial artist is a warrior who goes so far to help they will risk their very welfare and life just because they can. Not because they view this is expected of them.

Conversely, the coward helps as part of an agenda. A coward keeps track of his 'good deeds' because he expects to get something in return and, predictably, turns on their "friends" when those expectations are not met.

A genuine martial artist finds it a pleasure to give for the sake of giving, where a coward likes it only as opportunity, to benefit.

When was the last time somebody reached out to you for help? Was there the slightest bit of reluctancy? Felt the slightest bit of rejection towards either the person or his request? Then your coward played you! Even if you complied, eventually.

8. Be generous!

A genuine martial artist gives their everything because there exists no fear of depletion nor does one need energy to uphold anything. Everything the martial artist has to offer is made available. Sharing resources: financial, emotional, intellectual, or physical.

Have you ever caught yourself trying to give less than you really have and justifying that behavior, even manipulating the truth to make your actions look sincere?

9. Be ruthlessly dangerous to be kind.

Restraint and mercy can only happen in being in a position of power. That only happens when you are capable of being ruthless.

A good man is a man capable of great violence that keeps evil at bay.

In conclusion, be diligent in how you follow these "9 Tips" while also being self-conscious is next to impossible to be a martial artist, a warrior, can do it all the time.' By owning your inner coward, you become transformed, made unstoppable.

Frank Dux

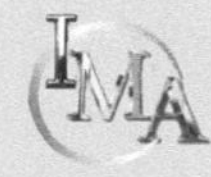

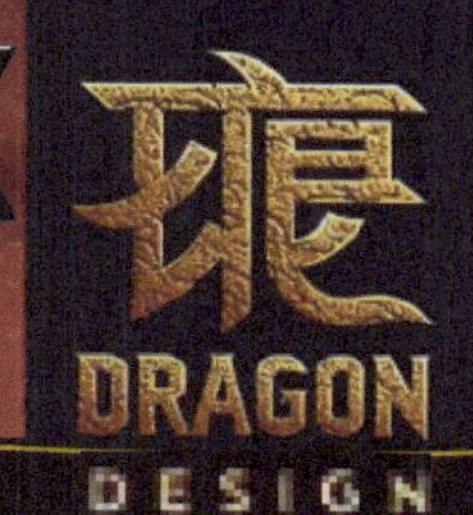

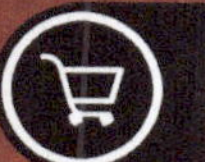

1 (725) 377 - 8092   **1 (725) 377 - 8092**

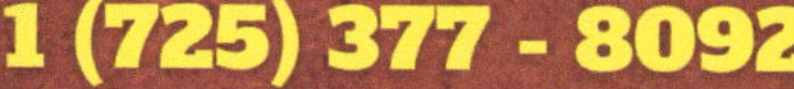

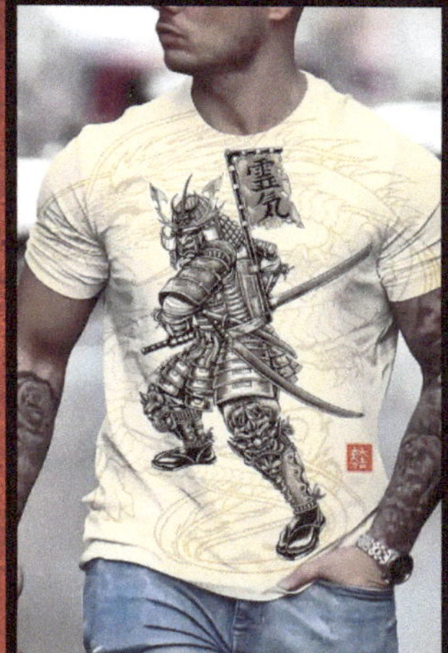
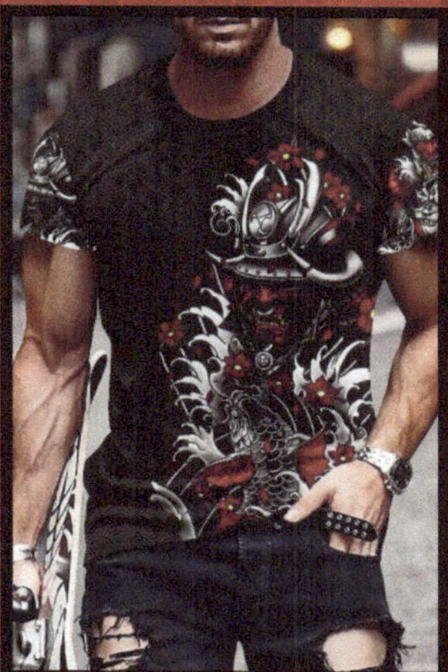
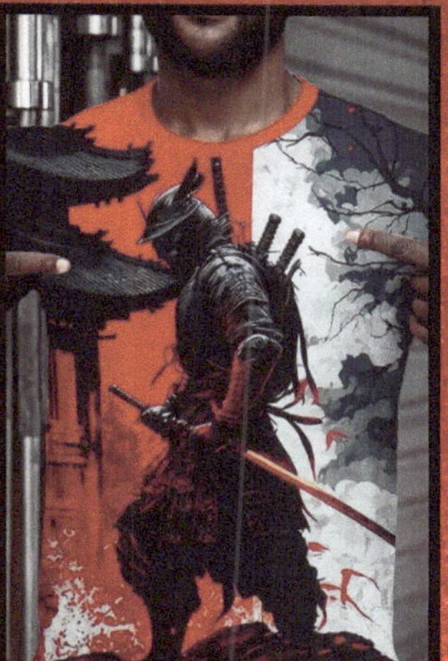
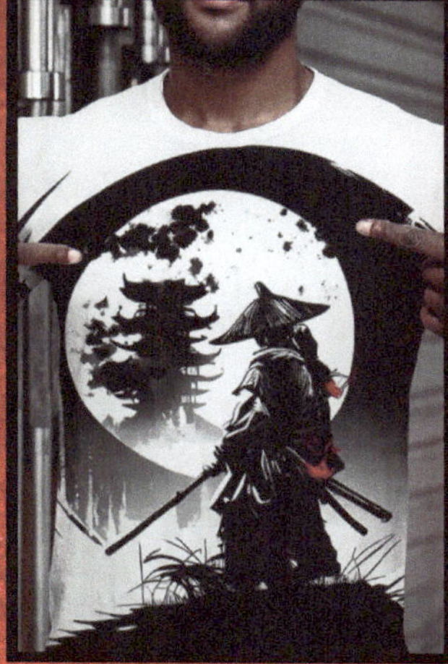

Biege	**Black**	**Black / Red**	**White / Blk**
$19.95 + S&H	$19.95 + S&H	$19.95 + S&H	$19.95 + S&H
Sizes S / M / L / XL / XXl		Sizes S / M / L / XL / XXl	

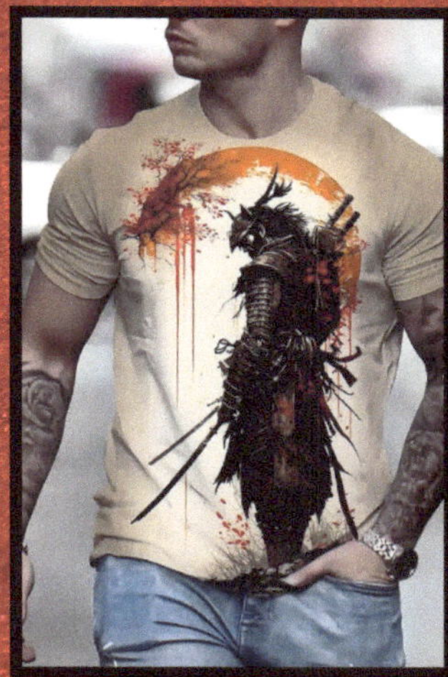
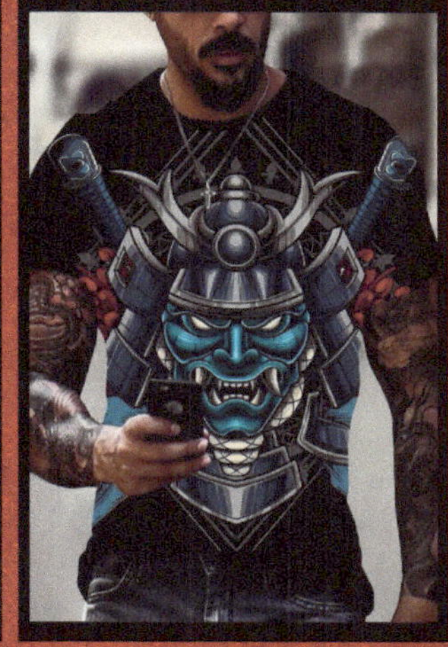
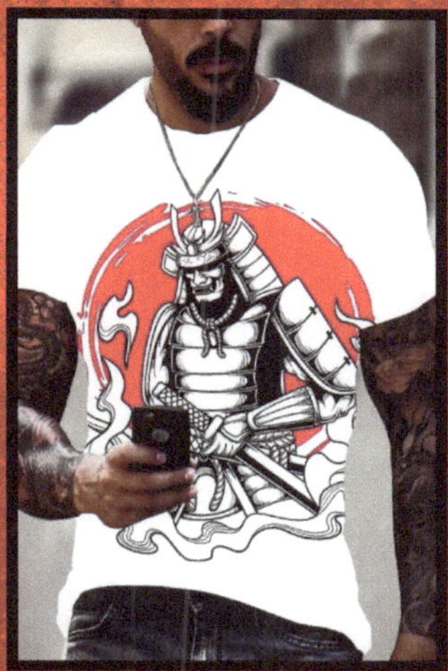
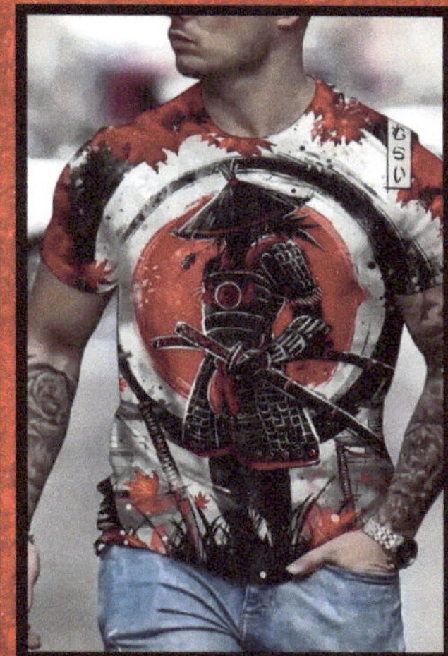

| **Biege** | **Blk / Grey** | **White / Red / Blk** | **Red / Black** |
| $19.95 + S&H | $19.95 + S&H | $19.95 + S&H | $19.95 + S&H |

NEW ARRIVAL SAMURAI GEAR

Dragonwearbranddesign@gmail.com

WHERE WE COME FROM

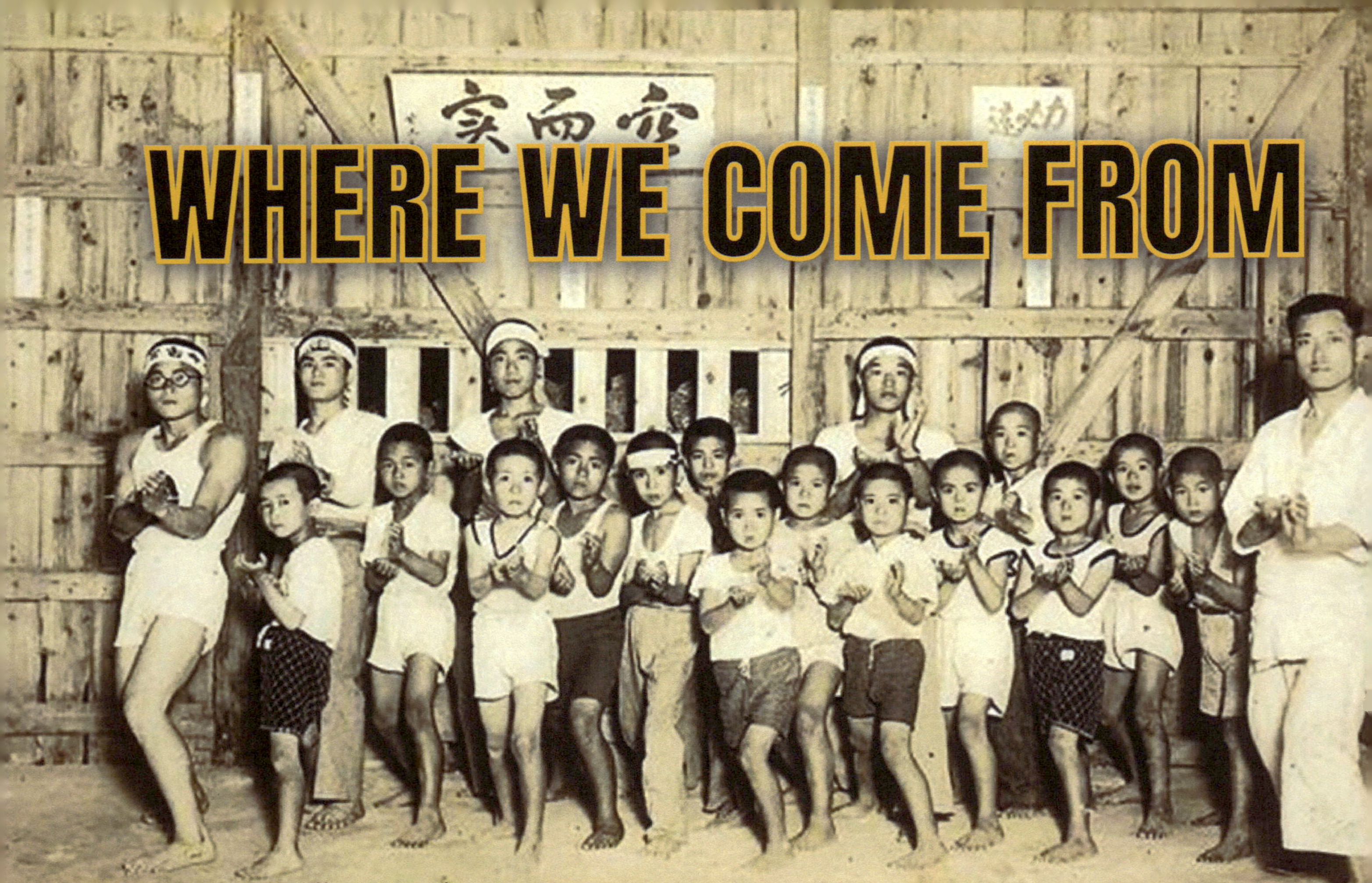

Written By Allen Woodman

I am not a Master nor a grandmaster of any art form or system. I do not even like or allow others to use that term with me. I have over 42 years training in the martial arts directly.

I have personally lived and trained in Asia and Japan for more than 20 of those years. Training in Japan at several of the top (Hombu) dojos was a delight and high honor.

Although it has been a great opportunity to have trained with such great teachers of traditional martial arts, I have never thought that the location of training was ever a real evaluation of skill and dedication.

I have only received my 6th Dan certificate after a rigorous belt test in Japan with no less than three higher ranking Black Belts from the school several years ago, just before my return to the USA.

When I was awarded my 6th Dan rank, I was told that I was one of a few that have attained the rank of 6th Dan. Of that, there were only around one hundred and twelve 6th Dans in all Japan at that time. Of those I was one of only fifteen foreigners to do so.

I was of course delighted to hear such news and noted to myself that I had accomplished much in my many years of study.

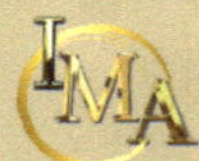

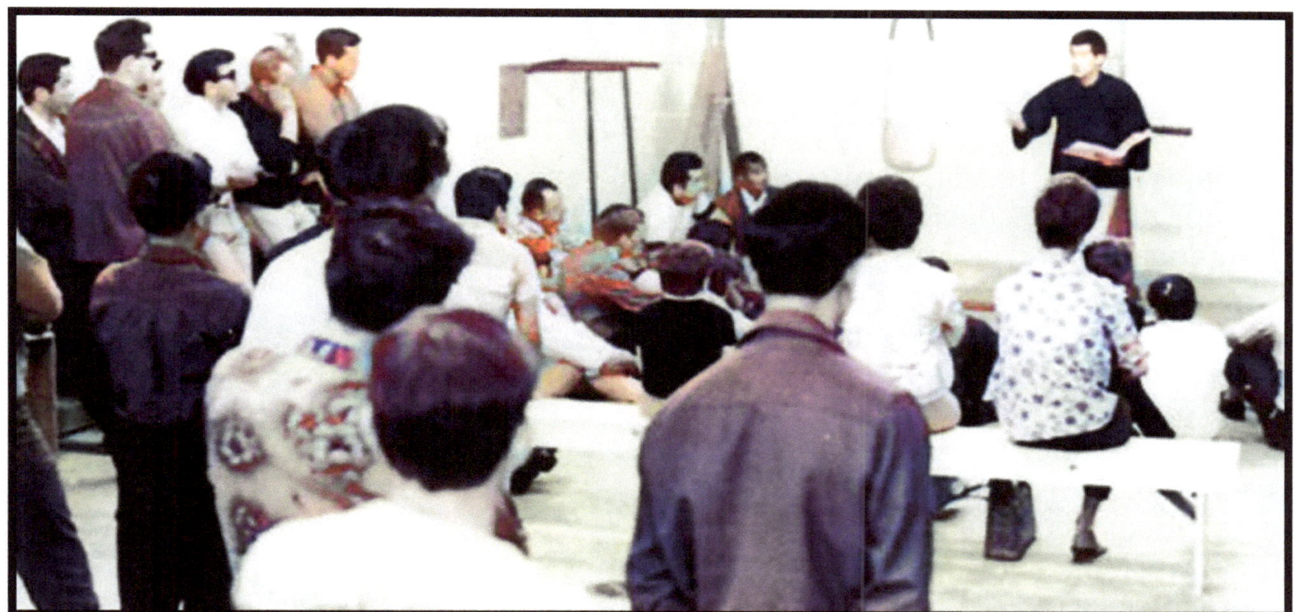

Growing up and training in Japan, it would have been an amazing sight to meet or even train with someone of the rank of 9th or God forbid even a 10th Dan.

As I reflect back, I cannot actually remember ever meeting in person, a 10th Dan instructor in Japan or China.

In Japan, Okinawa and China the orginal teachers never wore belts or graded students within levels of study. It was something that just was not needed. The teacher knew where each student was in their training.

There was an article in one of the Martial Arts magazines years ago, in which a high-ranking Black Belt (unspecified) from Okinawa visited the USA. He exclaimed, *"In all of Japan, there are but a handful of 10th Dans, yet in the NYC Yellow Pages, there are so many men with 10th Dans. The Martial Arts here must be very good!"*- He was being sarcastic.

Upon my return to the United States after a 14-year hiatus, I could not believe the multitudes of 10th Dan masters that I have encountered on my travels.

Some instructors claiming rather boastful ranks that upon demonstration and application would not be allowed a 1st Dan ranking in any school that I have ever trained in.

It's a sad statement that martial artist and students are hung up on rank levels and will believe that anyone can simply start their own system after a few years of training.

The term Soke (Founder or Father of a system) is so overused in America. In Asia I can't even remember the last time I even met a Soke. Here I only need walk three miles and I can hit ten or more.

The state of the martial arts in America is in decline.

I believe personally that the statement used by Bruce Lee, Founder of Jeet Kun DO (Way of the Intercepting Fist) "use what is useful" has been misused and propagated to a level and status in America beyond its intended reference.

When he made that statement, he was speaking to a group of dedicated martial artist that mostly already had their brown belts or black belts in other arts. These were students who attended classes regularly with Bruce lee. The Most active students had already learned the basics and the basis of martial arts within their respective martial arts training prior to their study with Bruce Lee.

However, just because you have trained in a martial art (even for several years) does not imply that you have mastered an art or system. "It takes more than a lifetime to master a single kata in a single level." O'Sensei Gichin Funakoshi (Founder of Shotokan Karate and Father of Traditional Japanese Karate today).

Yet, here in America we have so many masters that have begun their own styles and systems with less than 10-15 years training in various arts.

WAKE UP and smell the permeating decline of martial arts in America. We should not fall victim to Rank and Status. Training in the martial arts as a balance of life and fitness regimen should be our only suffice and conclusion of our time involved. Not as a way to boast yourself or to have others "kow tao" to our benevolence.

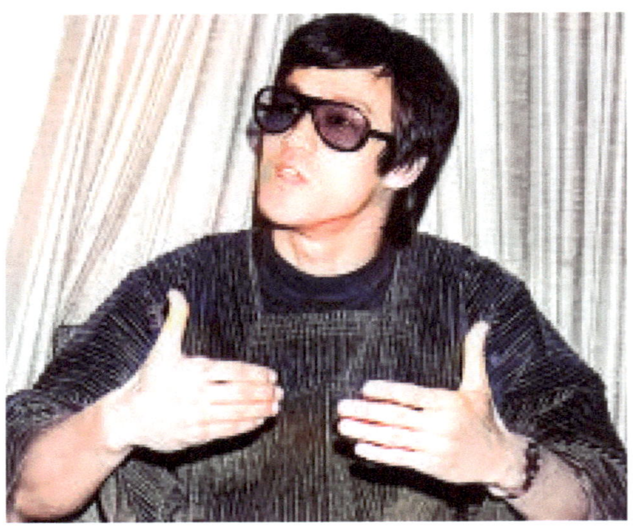

"use what is useful"
Bruce Lee

Some have misquoted that the great teacher Jigaro Kano (Born in 1860) started his own art of Judo at the age of 22. I'm sorry to say that O'Sensei Kano did not found Judo as a system of his own until 1898 which made him 48 years old at the time of its implementation of the art now known as Judo (Originally Jikinshin ryu Jujitsu).

This was after years of study in traditional Jujitsu under Master Fukuda and Master Fukushima (From the age of 14). Also, he had already been the Professor of the prestigious Tokyo Imperial University in Japan (Professor of Physiology) and later became Minister of Education in the same year he began to teach Judo as a Rentai Ho (Physical exercise) Shobu Ho (MartialArt) and Shushin Ho (Cultivation of wisdom).

History is in the details, ladies and gentleman. Professor Kano never took a 10th Dan title. However, he was the person solely named as the inventor of the Kyu grading system within belt ranks that we all use today.

Kano, gave before his death the only10th Dan ever given to that point to his student Sensei Kyuzo Mifune. To ensure that there would be no disputes amongst his followers as to whom would oversee the Kodokan Dojo and the art of Judo's future.

A recent question was asked of me in a forum that found quit interesting and was a well-founded query.

"Why can't there be Master and grandmaster in America?

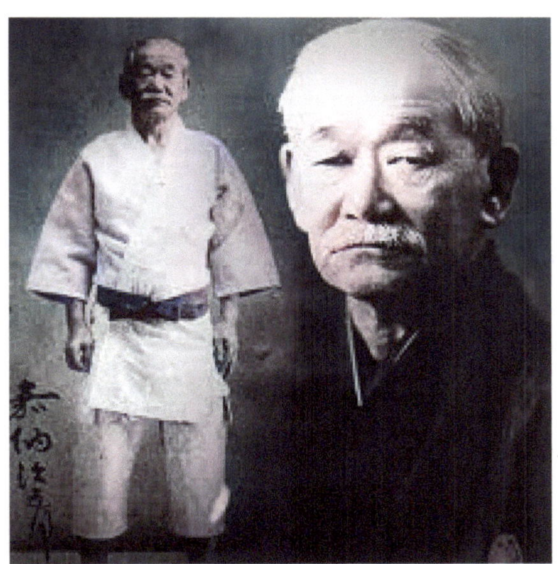

"Se Ryoko Zenyo Jita Kyoe'."
Train in the arts to honor your
country and your community

O'Sensei JigaroKano .

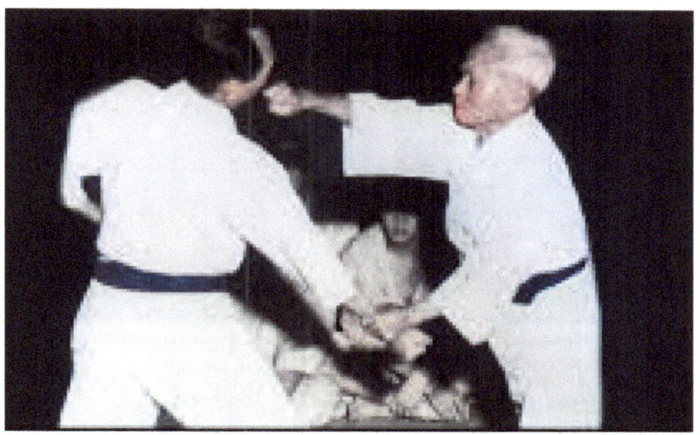

It takes more than a lifetime to master
a single kata in a single level."

O'Sensei Gichin Funakoshi

Since there have been Martial Arts in America for more than 60+ years."

In Asia there are actually ministries (Such as the Japanese Butokukai) that oversee the authority and certification of all Black Belts. It also permits and registers or disallows schools to be opened in cities throughout Japan or not. A registry that cannot be denied of lineage.

This makes it actually impossible or more improbable for anyone to declare themselves a master or rank that they have not actually been certified to.

Martial Arts in America has been around since the early 1900's (references to Jujitsu in printed book form can be found circa 1904).

Back in 1904, President Theodore "Teddy" Roosevelt practiced judo and jujitsu three afternoons a week, using a ground floor office in the White House as his workout space.

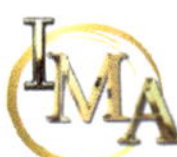

Commercial martial arts were not openly taught until after WW2, when was it opened to the general public to study. Mostly it was returning G.I.s that had studied in Japan and Asia for a few years in their respective arts.

Since then, there was merely a handful in the scheme of populace that actually helped build martial arts throughout the USA.

In the early 1960's there was a boom in both schools and proliferation of martial arts in America.

That is the point of most inception to martial arts here in the USA. So, when others begin referring to martial arts being 60+ years, it was at this high point that many began their journey. From here students began to experience the arts in its basic element.

I say basic because, the individuals that were teaching were not of high level at that time. The understanding of study was somewhat limited and slow paced for students. Training and understanding were slow, therefore many students did not stay in a single school or dojo.

Even the great Robert Trias (Shuri Karate) Instructor and owner of the very first recorded martial arts school in the USA in 1946, was not even a 6th Dan until the mid-1980's).

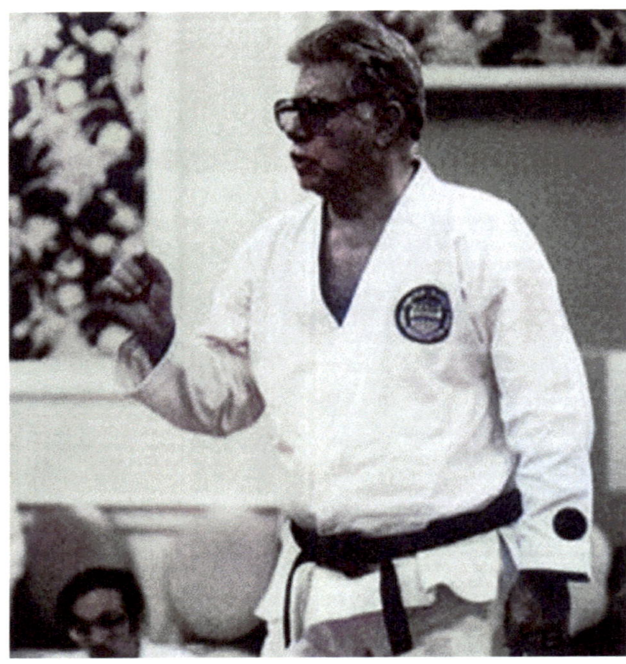

Sensei Robert Trias - Photo circa 1975

Therefore, any students training under Master Trias would not have been able to promote past the rank of 4th Dan until that time (1980's).

Martial students began searching elsewhere for answers and became wandering Ronin (Master-less Warriors). Until more formal schools began opening and expanding in the early 1970's.

In Asia the martial arts as a whole are ingrained within the societal culture. Within the history and formality of etiquette that all natively raised Asians are taught from childhood. This does allow them to devote their understanding of the arts a bit faster than most foreigners because they have no necessity to study the language and etiquette of their own cultural background.

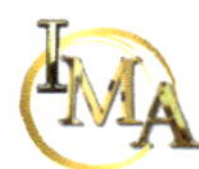

There are so many facets to the history of martial arts in America that it is hard to establish a clear timeline from this point.

There have been very few schools that have survived and are still in operation today that began further back than the 1980's. Whereas in Japan and Asia schools have records that establish themselves and their specific lineage that date over 500 years or more.

So, to answer the question "Why can't there be Masters and Grandmasters in the arts here in America?"

The answer is that the statement of 60+ years actually can only be boiled down to less than 40 years in actuality.

That would still be more than adequate time to create Master level instructors, IF they ALL had begun then, and stayed within that single art or system since, without long or prolonged breaks in training and study.

The sheer number of Master and Grandmasters far outweigh the number of certified students at the founding schools.

Since America does not yet have an official or even self-imposed authority over certification of martial arts it's hard to know whom to trust and who is a true master upon a glance.

A good student of martial arts made a statement and proffers a few true questions we should all ask ourselves and those around us. These questions and statements I felt were the truest understanding of rank that I have heard in many years.

<u>Glenn Perry</u> wrote …
"This is a current topic of SERIOUS discussion in many martial arts forums. The situation exists in the United States for a multitude of reasons, and some are truly valid. First, I would point out that Japan/Okinawa are lands of martial arts traditions probably not as open to change and innovation like what is found and acceptable in the USA.

Martial arts have been in North America for over 100 years and has evolved and continues to permeate into our Western culture."

He continues with… *"Are we dealing with a situation of over inflated rank and misrepresentation of martial arts titles YES! Are the martial arts in the US operating under the same guidelines that influence age, time, grade, one's personal skill level and accomplish-ments, contributions and giving back to the martial arts community, etc., as the guidelines and measuring sticks being use in Japan and Okinawa?*

I'm not sure, but I don't think so!!

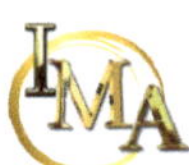

I am left with the question, how is it possible for someone to claim at 25 or 30 years of age to be a Grandmaster, Soke and founder of a martial arts style during peacetime study?

Our arts don't have switches turning on and off when we put on and take of our uniform!

This way of life is to be lived first and there are no short cuts! The belt, whatever color, is made of cotton and is symbolic of something much more meaningful than rank....

"Walk a single path, becoming neither cocky with victory nor broken with defeat, without forgetting caution when all is quiet or becoming frightened when danger threatens."
- O'Sensei Jigaro Kano

These final statements I must admit are a strong cast of martial artists thinking. However, I believe they are truer to the nature of the questions we seek in our training.

I would not deem myself educated enough to know which is correct, or which is improper. I can only state that martial arts have never been about rank or status. It should never be the goal to attain some title given by some random group attesting to your skill level.

In my humble opinion, I can only ask this question?

What did that Founding father of whatever American mixed martial arts system they created FIND?

What did they create that was not there before them. In other arts such as Judo, Aikido and some systems of karate, the founders created a new path, a unique delivery of already exposed movements and ability. By simply mixing systems and styles does not imply an individual creation.

Some new stated founders have simply mixed or applied pieces of other already formed systems or styles and grabbed portions therein as if the martial arts were a holloween candy grab bag.

Some principles an dfoundations do not work together conducively. Some arts are rooted in form while others are more sport attentive and remain light on their feet. Ho wcan these co-exist?

I have no clear understanding no answers. I only ask questions that should be apperent to anyone with a basic understanding.

The proof is in the pudding as the saying goes.

"The answers are all on the dojo floor."
- Shihan Allen Woodman.

Allen Woodman

HISTORY OF JAPANESE MARTIAL ARTS

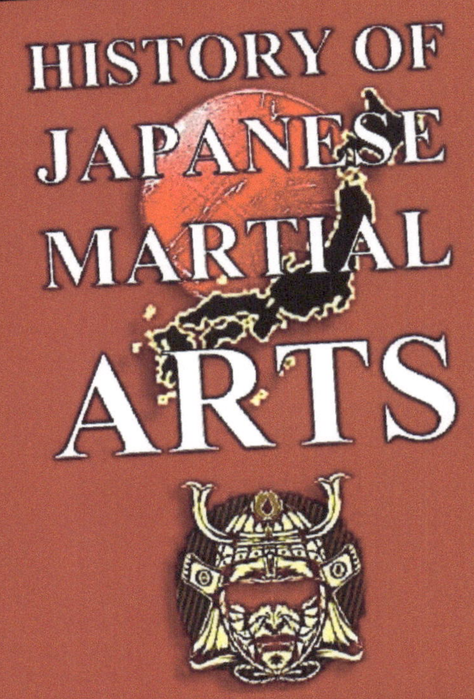

⭐⭐⭐⭐⭐ <u>Stu Rose</u>

As a Martial Arts Instructor for over 25 yrs. I found this to be a very good book I enjoyed reading it. I know a fair amount of history but this book filled in a lot history I didn't know but always wanted to. I highly recommend it for martial artists at any level who want to learn about the roots of various Japanese styles and personalities i.e. karate, Jujitsu, Judo, etc.

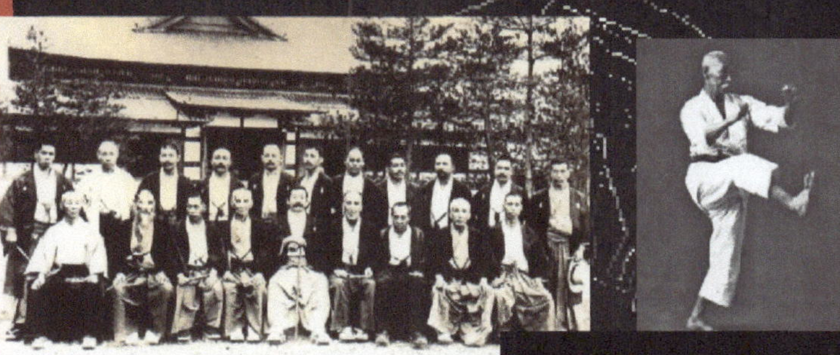

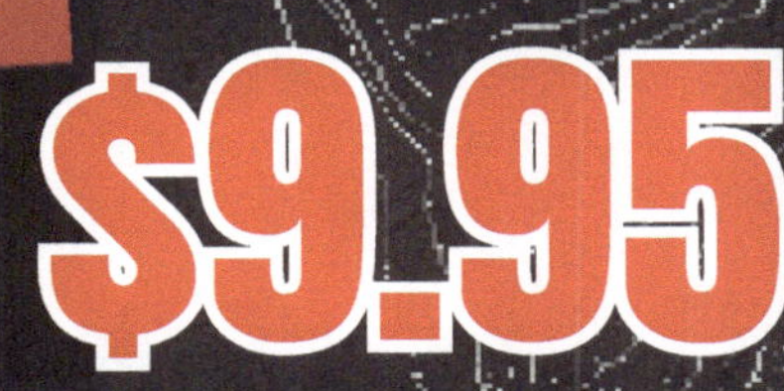

$9.95

Turn of the century 1900`s Japan. Many people were turning toward the western ways and progressing toward a more united front. In the midst of all this change came many great teachers of Martial arts. Aikido, Judo, Jujitsu and Karate in its many forms all started in Japan. These Arts are thriving in society today due to the rigid adherence of Japanese culture and tradition. Shihan Allen Woodman has spent nearly 40 years training in multiple forms of martial arts with 20 years training in Japan. A certified 6th degree black belt, he has devoted his life to learning the many facets that comprise traditional Japanese martial arts of Aikido, Karate, Judo, Karate and Jujitsu. Reading this book will give you a better understanding of the beginnings of all traditional Japanese martial arts from a unique perspective. Learn the foundation of the traditional arts, who started them and why."

Allen Woodman is a learned person with such a vast knowledge of the true history of the arts it would be foolish of any one not to listen to his stories

"Michael Matsuda, Curator, Martial Arts History Museum

AVAILABLE ON AMAZON.COM

SUMIKO NAKANO
THE SILENT LIONESS

In the world of Mixed Martial Arts (MMA), where strength and aggression often dominate, Sumiko Nakano stands out not just for her skill, but for her silent strength and resilience.

Known in the MMA community as "The Silent Lioness," Sumiko has carved out a unique path that blends modern combat sports with ancient martial traditions. This article delves into her journey, highlighting the personal experiences that shaped her, the traditional arts that ground her, and her vision for the future.

Family History and Cultural Heritage Sumiko Nakano's family history is a cornerstone of her identity and deeply influences her martial arts and literary pursuits.

She is related to Nakano Takeko, a legendary onna musha (female warrior) who fought valiantly during the Boshin War. Nakano Takeko is Sumiko's first cousin four times removed, and her legacy of courage and honor is something Sumiko strives to embody in her own life.

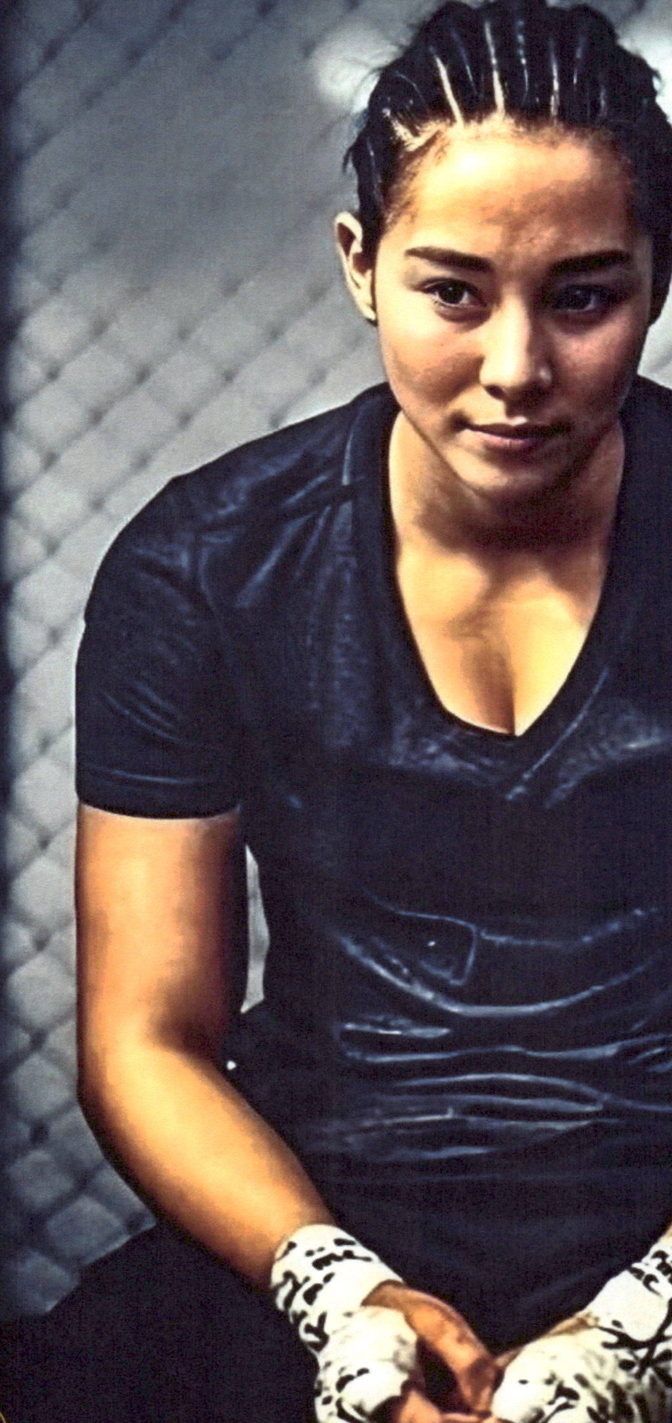

Sumiko sees herself as a modern onna musha, adhering to the old Japanese traditions and the Bushido code.

This code, emphasizing virtues such as honor, courage, and loyalty, guides her actions both in and out of the ring. Her dedication to martial arts is not just about physical training but also about upholding these timeless principles.

Growing up, Sumiko was immersed in the stories of her ancestors. The tale of Nakano Takeko, who led her fellow women warriors with unmatched bravery, left a profound impact on her. Her spirit lives on in Sumiko's practice and daily life, inspiring her to pursue excellence and uphold the values Nakano Takeko cherished.

This rich heritage has instilled in Sumiko a sense of responsibility to honor her ancestors through her actions, both in the martial arts arena and beyond.

Sumiko was born in Osaka, Japan. Her martial arts journey began almost as soon as she could walk. At the tender age of four, she started training in Taekwondo, a discipline that would lay the foundation for her striking techniques and agility. Just a year later, she was introduced to Naginatajutsu, an ancient Japanese martial art that would deeply influence her philosophy and approach to combat.

These early experiences were not just about physical training but also about instilling a sense of discipline, respect, and connection to her cultural heritage.

After a tragic car accident when Sumiko was three, she lost her parents and her ability to speak, rendering her mute.

Following the accident, she was adopted and moved to the UK. Despite this upheaval, Sumiko spent two months every year with her grandparents in Osaka, where she received training in Naginatajutsu, Kenjutsu, and Karate. These visits were crucial in maintaining her connection to her Japanese roots and heritage.

In the UK, Sumiko balanced her time between rigorous martial arts training and her academic pursuits. Despite facing the challenge of being mute, she excelled in her studies, attending prestigious institutions like Boundary Oak School and Fareham College.

Her educational journey culminated in an LLB Bachelor of Laws from the University of London, and she is currently expanding her legal expertise with a Master's in International Business Law at the University of Liverpool. These academic achievements reflect her commitment to continuous learning and personal growth, mirroring her dedication in the dojo.

One of the most defining aspects of Sumiko's journey has been living with a speech disability. As a result of the car accident, Sumiko cannot speak at all. This challenge has profoundly shaped her life and career, teaching her invaluable lessons about communication, perseverance, and strength.

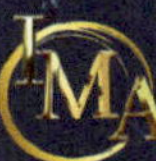

From a young age, she had to find alternative ways to express herself, relying on actions rather than words. This reliance on non-verbal communication has greatly influenced her approach to martial arts, where every move and gesture carries meaning.

The nickname "The Silent Lioness" is a testament to Sumiko's silent strength. In a sport where trash talk and loud bravado are common, she has chosen to let her skills speak for themselves. Her silence in the ring is not a weakness but a source of power. It allows her to focus entirely on her performance, using every ounce of her energy to execute techniques with precision and grace. This approach has become a defining characteristic of her fighting style.

Several vital milestones distinguish Sumiko's martial arts career. She has earned brown belts in Brazilian Jiu-Jitsu and Kickboxing, a 1st Dan black belt in Taekwondo, and a 3rd Dan in Naginatajutsu. Each of these achievements represents years of dedication and countless hours of training. Brazilian Jiu-Jitsu, emphasizing grappling and submission, has honed her ground game, while Kickboxing has added power and precision to her striking.

Training in Kenjutsu has refined Sumiko's combat skills, teaching her the importance of timing and accuracy. This blend of traditional and modern martial arts has made her a versatile and unpredictable fighter, capable of adapting to any situation in the octagon.

While she continues to train in Muay Thai and Karate, these disciplines complement her existing skills, adding layers of complexity to her fighting style.
Personal Stories of Resilience and Dedication

Sumiko's journey is filled with personal stories that showcase her resilience and dedication. For instance, her time spent training with her grandparents in Osaka was not just about honing her skills but also about connecting deeply with her heritage.

 The discipline and techniques she learned during these summer visits have impacted her martial arts journey.

Another significant experience was overcoming the challenges posed by her speech disability. Sumiko has demonstrated that communication goes beyond words, using her actions and achievements to inspire others.

Looking ahead, Sumiko's goals are as ambitious as they are inspiring. She aims to continue developing her skills in martial arts, pushing the boundaries of what she can achieve. She also plans to share her knowledge through teaching and exhibitions, hoping to inspire the next generation of martial artists.

The primary message Sumiko wishes to convey through her journey is the power of resilience and silent strength.

Despite facing significant adversities, such as the loss of her parents and her speech disability, she has found ways to communicate and excel through martial arts and writing.

Her story is a testament to the fact that challenges can be transformed into strengths and that one's voice can manifest powerfully through actions and perseverance.

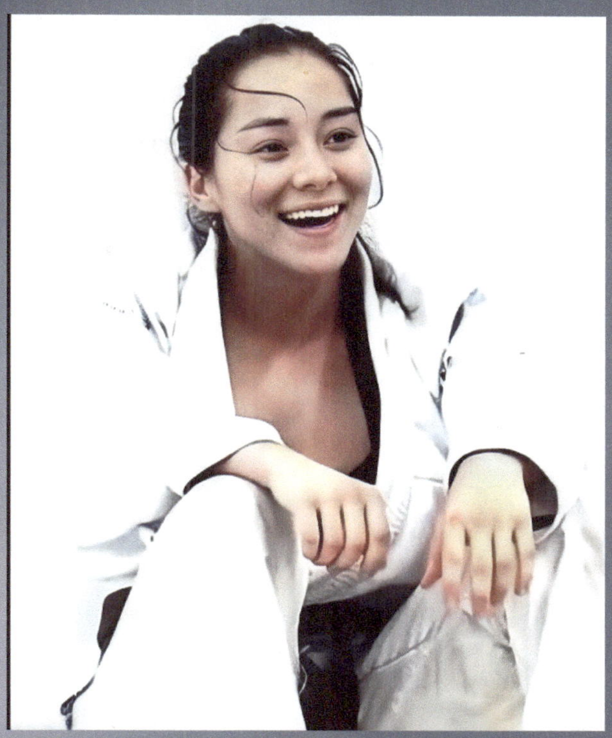

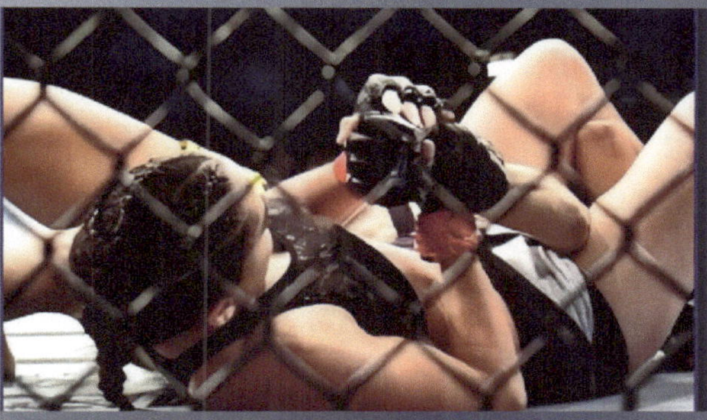

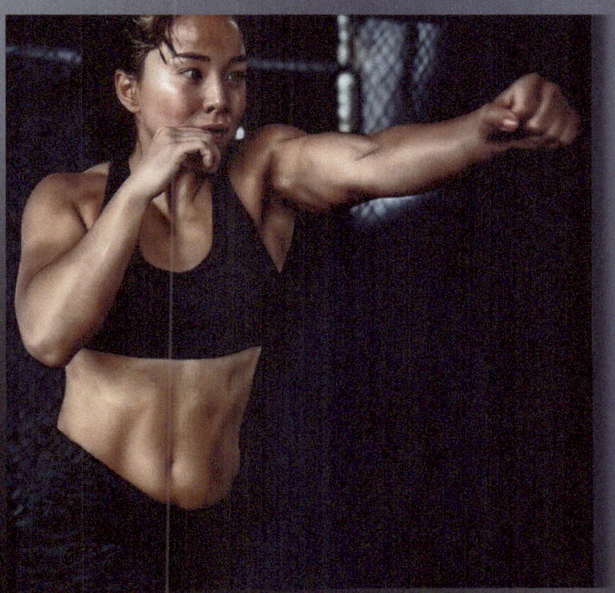

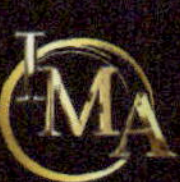

Sumiko Nakano's journey from traditional martial arts to the competitive world of MMA is a story of resilience, dedication, and silent strength. Her achievements, both in the dojo and the octagon, are a testament to her unwavering determination and passion for martial arts.

As she continues to pursue her goals and inspire others through her story, Sumiko embodies the spirit of a true warrior, demonstrating that the greatest strength often lies in silence and perseverance.

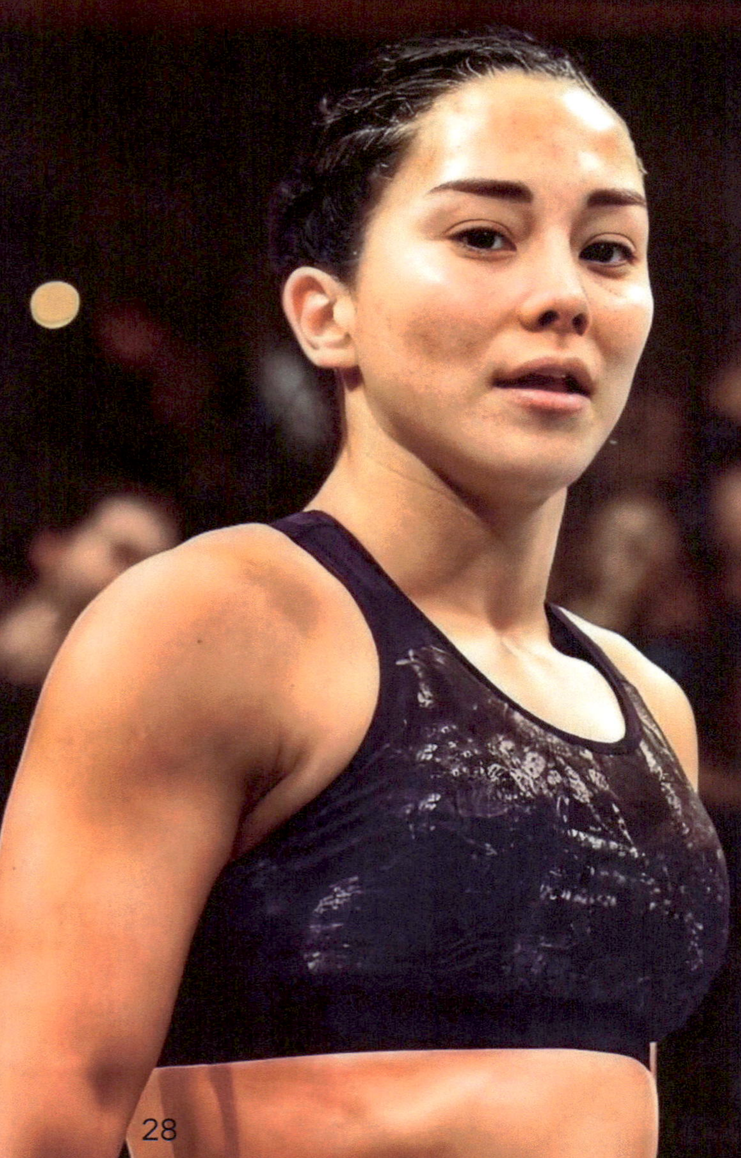

Sumiko Nakano's life is a fascinating blend of two worlds—Osaka, Japan, and London, United Kingdom—each contributing uniquely to her growth and success. She immerses herself in a culture deeply rooted in tradition and discipline in Japan.

Osaka's serene landscapes and historic dojos provide the perfect backdrop for her rigorous training in Naginatajutsu, Kenjutsu, and Shotokan Karate. Here, the ancient Bushido code of honor, courage, and loyalty is not just a concept but a way of life.

These experiences are integral to her development as a martial artist, connecting her to her ancestral roots and reinforcing the principles that guide her actions.

Sumiko is also involved in her traditional family business in Japan. This aspect of her life adds a layer of intrigue as she honors her family's legacy through endeavors that require the same discipline and dedication she brings to her training. The nature of this business reflects the deep respect and commitment Sumiko holds for her heritage and the values passed down through generations.

In stark contrast, London offers Sumiko a dynamic and diverse environment. The city's vibrant energy and modern outlook have broadened her horizons, allowing her to balance her martial arts training with academic pursuits.

The state-of-the-art training facilities and the support of a diverse network of peers and mentors make London the perfect place for her to hone her skills and push her boundaries.

Life in London also allows her to experience a rich tapestry of cultures, cuisines, and arts, further enriching her personal and professional life. She embraces the city's fast pace and endless opportunities, finding inspiration in its blend of history and innovation.

Sumiko Nakano is a formidable martial artist, and in addition to her martial arts pursuits, she is also an accomplished author.

She has published several works that weave historical events with imaginative storytelling. Her book "Shadows of the Naginata" delves into the life of a young warrior in feudal Japan, drawing heavily from her own experiences and family history. Meanwhile, her series "Daughters of Wars: The Birth of Steel and Vengeance" explores the untold stories of women warriors, celebrating their strength and resilience.

Through her writing, she aims to inspire others, particularly those facing similar challenges, and highlight the importance of resilience and cultural heritage.

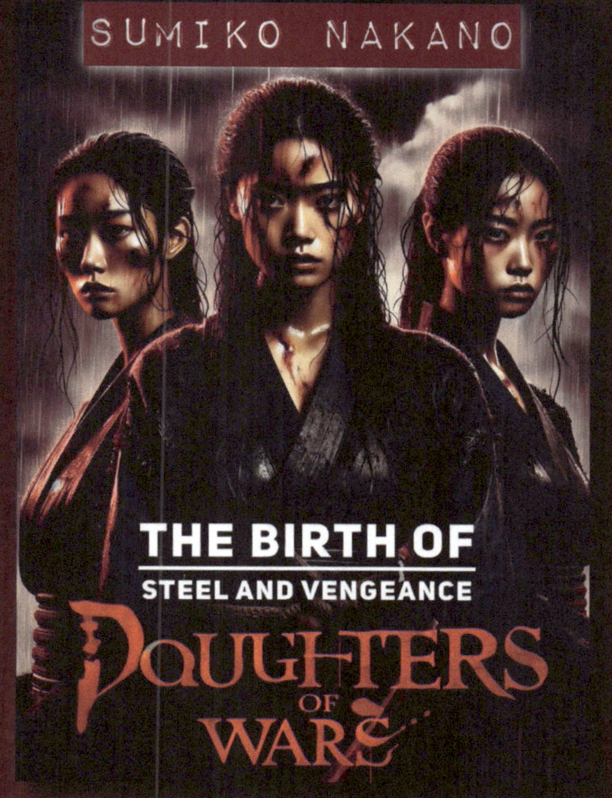

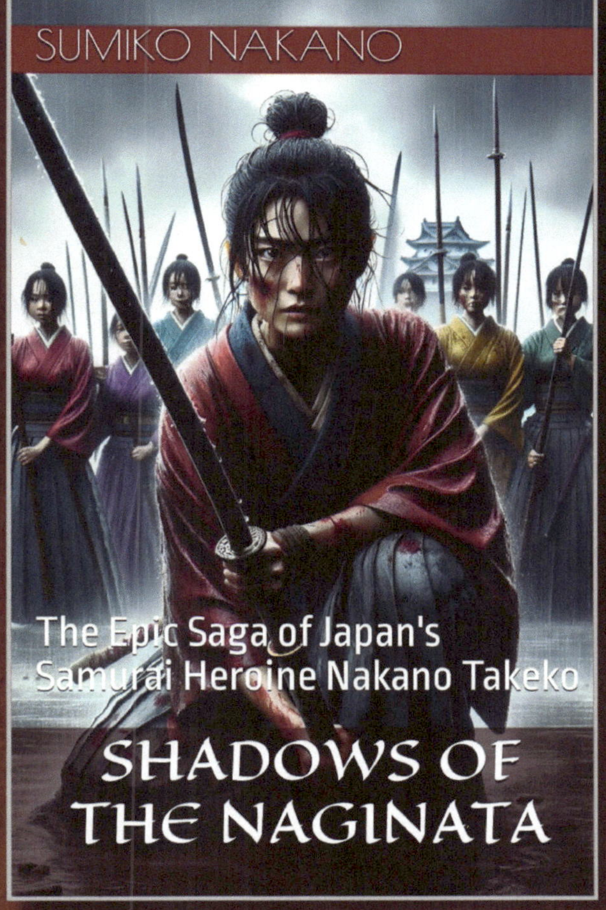

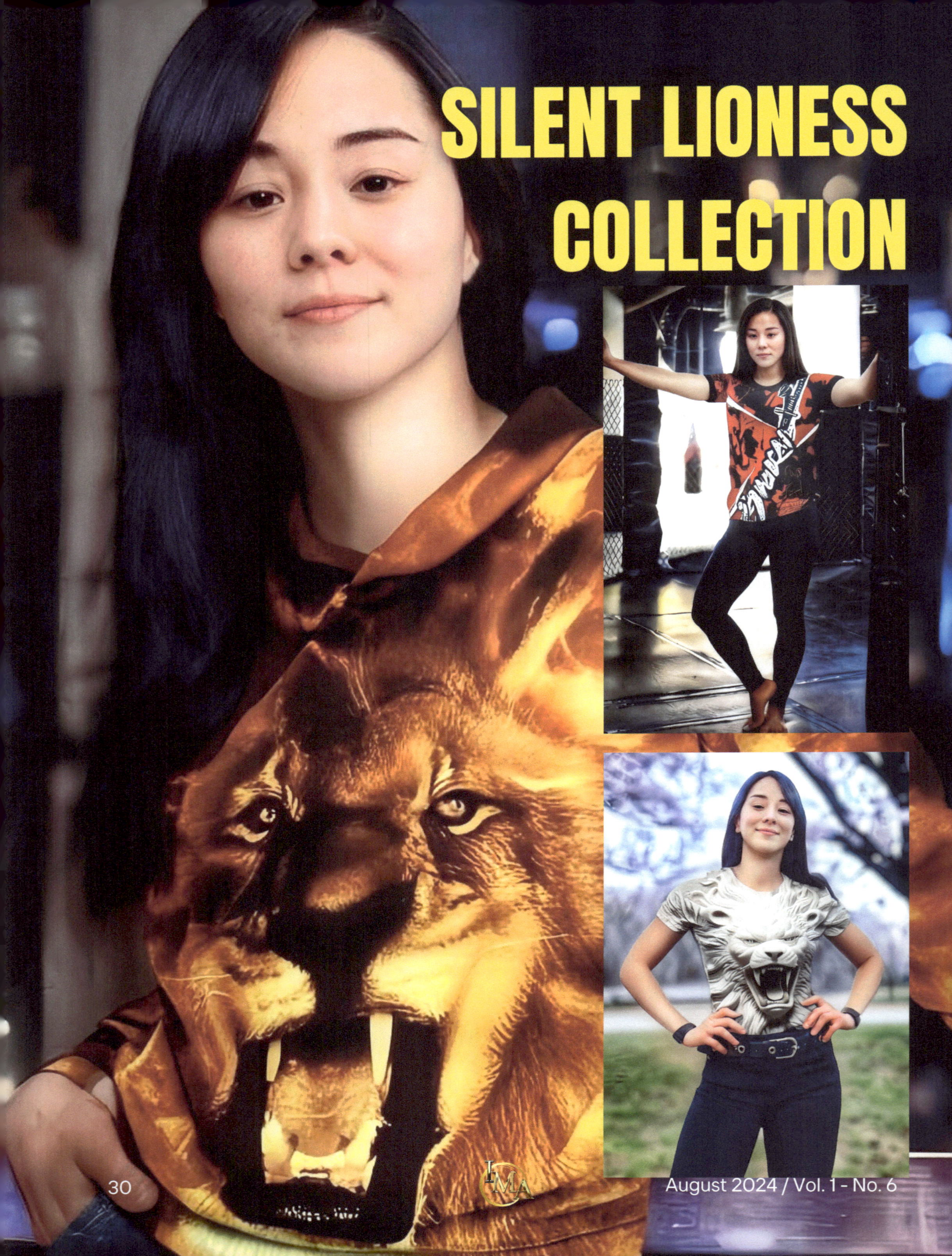

SILENT LIONESS
COLLECTION

Sumiko is also excited to introduce her new clothing line, the Lioness Collection, in partnership with Dragonwear Brand Designs.

This collaboration brings together her passion for martial arts and her love for fashion, resulting in a unique line of athletic and casual wear. Each piece in the Lioness Collection is designed to embody the strength, resilience, and grace that Sumiko represents both in and out of the dojo.

The Lioness Collection features a range of products, from stylish casual wear to comfortable everyday pieces, all crafted with the highest quality materials. The designs are inspired by Sumiko's own journey and the symbolism of the lioness—powerful, graceful, and fiercely protective.

Working with Dragonwear Brand, known for their innovative and stylish casual wear, has been an incredible experience for Sumiko. She is thrilled to share these designs with the world, hoping to inspire confidence and empowerment in everyone who wears them.

Future Aspirations

Looking to the future, Sumiko Nakano envisions continuing her evolution as both a martial artist and a writer. Over the next years, she plans to refine her skills across various martial arts disciplines and expand her literary portfolio with more captivating stories. Her goal is to explore new creative ventures and contribute positively to the worlds of martial arts and literature.

Sumiko's journey is a testament to the power of resilience, dedication, and silent strength—showing that with these qualities, any obstacle can be overcome and dreams can be realized.

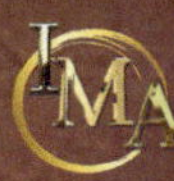

APACHE KNIFE COMBAT

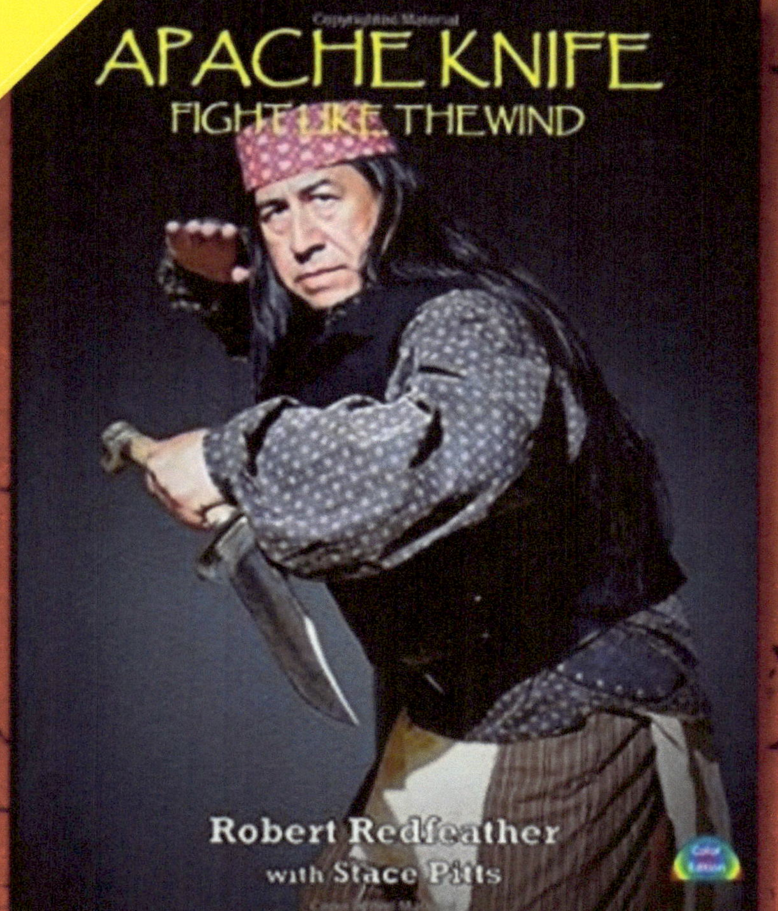

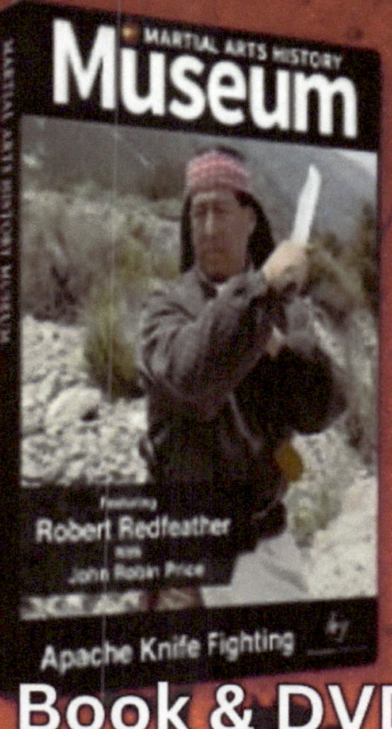

Book & DVD

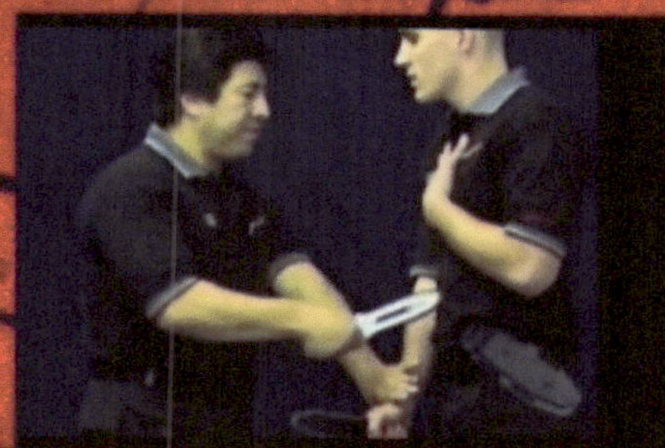

AVAILABLE NOW $49.95

Robert Redfeather's Apache Knife Combat System is a comprehensive knife fighting system that covers Apache history; close quarters combat techniques, defensive skills, respect for a knife and the value of human life. Apache knife is different, it does not teach you to stand your ground but to be fluid like the wind. "I am proud to keep alive a near extinct fighting art and Apache culture that values life as well as defensive techniques and skill. As my Apache Knife Combat System has become known, I have had more Native Americans seek me out to learn the fighting style of their ancestors. I am honored to have had the opportunity to plant this seed that has been hidden away and continue to watch it grow. I am so filled with pride to be teaching one of the oldest traditional Native American Fighting Arts."
- Robert Redfeather.

Redfeather teaches Law Enforcement, U.S. Military, private contractors as well as personal training for civilians.

This book is an introduction to basic Apache Knife® Combat System.

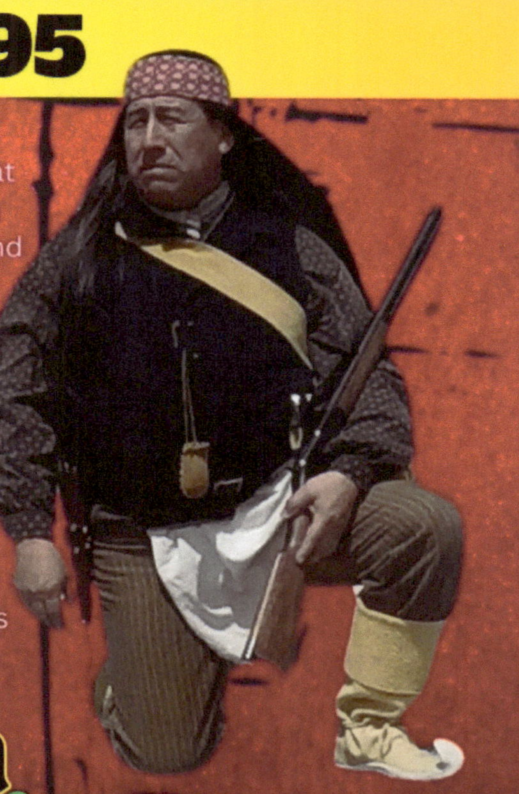

AVAILABLE ON AMAZON.COM

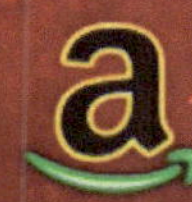

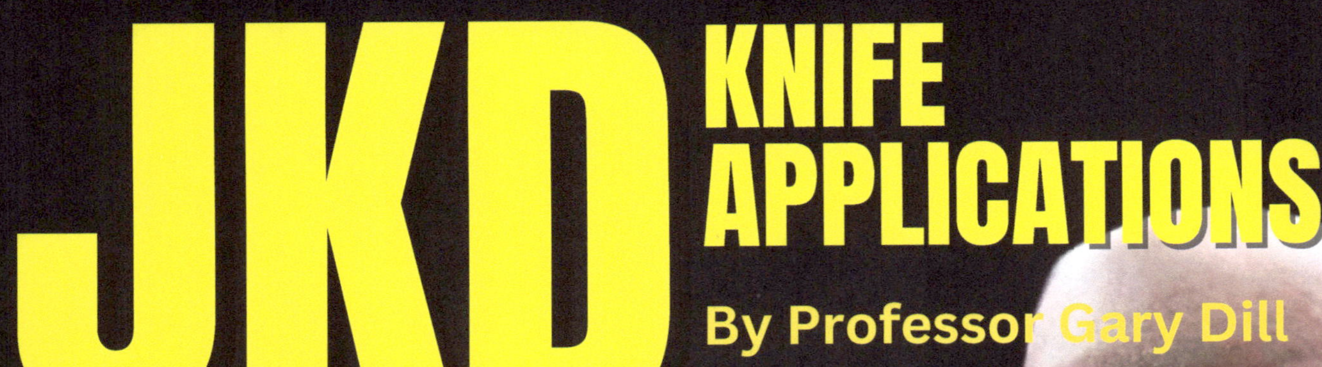

The knife has been vital to a warrior's personal arsenal for thousands of years.

It is nearly as old as mankind. Even with the high-tech weapons used in combat, the knife is still found in the hands of today's modern military combatant. In close-quarters combat, the blade is as important now as it was during the time of the ancient samurai.

Several years ago, the army announced that it was replacing traditional bayonet training (using the blade on the end of the rifle) with using the bayonet as a knife for CQC applications.

The knife has one purpose: to incapacitate or terminate the enemy.

For the combatant to be effective in using the knife, he/she must have two major components:

(1) the instinct to survive and the willingness to wound or terminate the enemy, and

(2) a realistic system of using the knife.

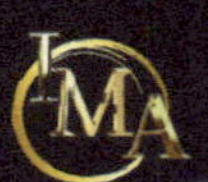

After returning from a tour of duty in Vietnam in early 1971, I was accepted in the exclusive Oakland JKD class taught by James Lee with Bruce Lee being the head instructor.

Regarding training with a knife, James told me that, "When you learn JKD, you already know how to use a knife. The knife becomes an extension of your hand. You simply do the same empty hand JKD techniques but, with the knife in your hand."

I then understood the principle of the Oakland JKD knife fighting, which was not related to Filipino Kali, Escrima, or any other knife fighting style, but was a different system of its own, based strictly on Bruce Lee's original Jeet Kune Do empty hand fighting techniques.

This laid the groundwork for my personal JKD combat knife system that I have been teaching for years. Just weeks after 9/11 I was hired by a military contractor company to develop a CQC empty hand and weapons program. Later a Homeland Security training company contracted me to provide them a CQC program to be taught to their members and clients. Since that time, I have trained many Homeland Security and Special Operation military personnel my system of JKD knife tactics.

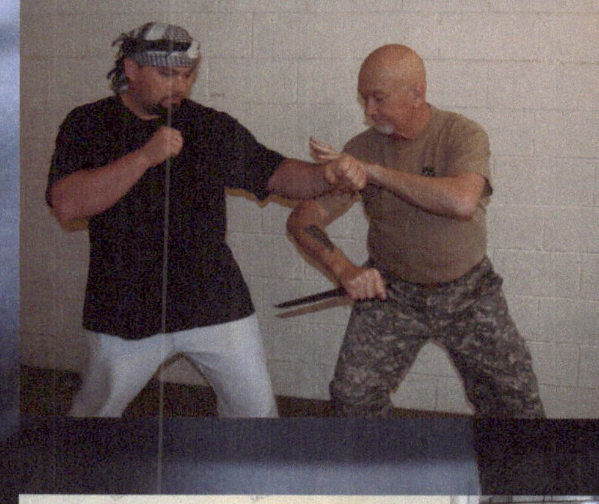

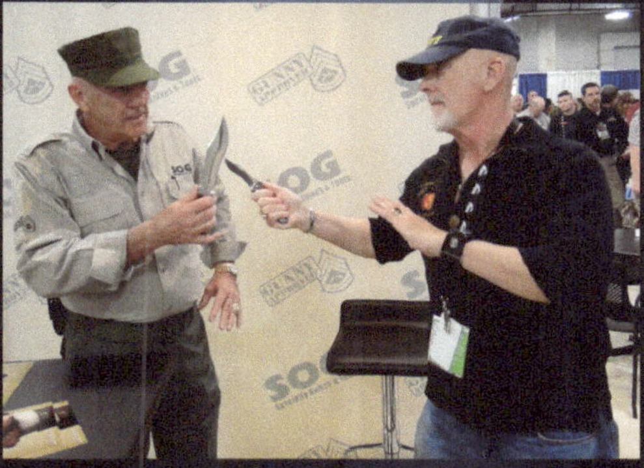

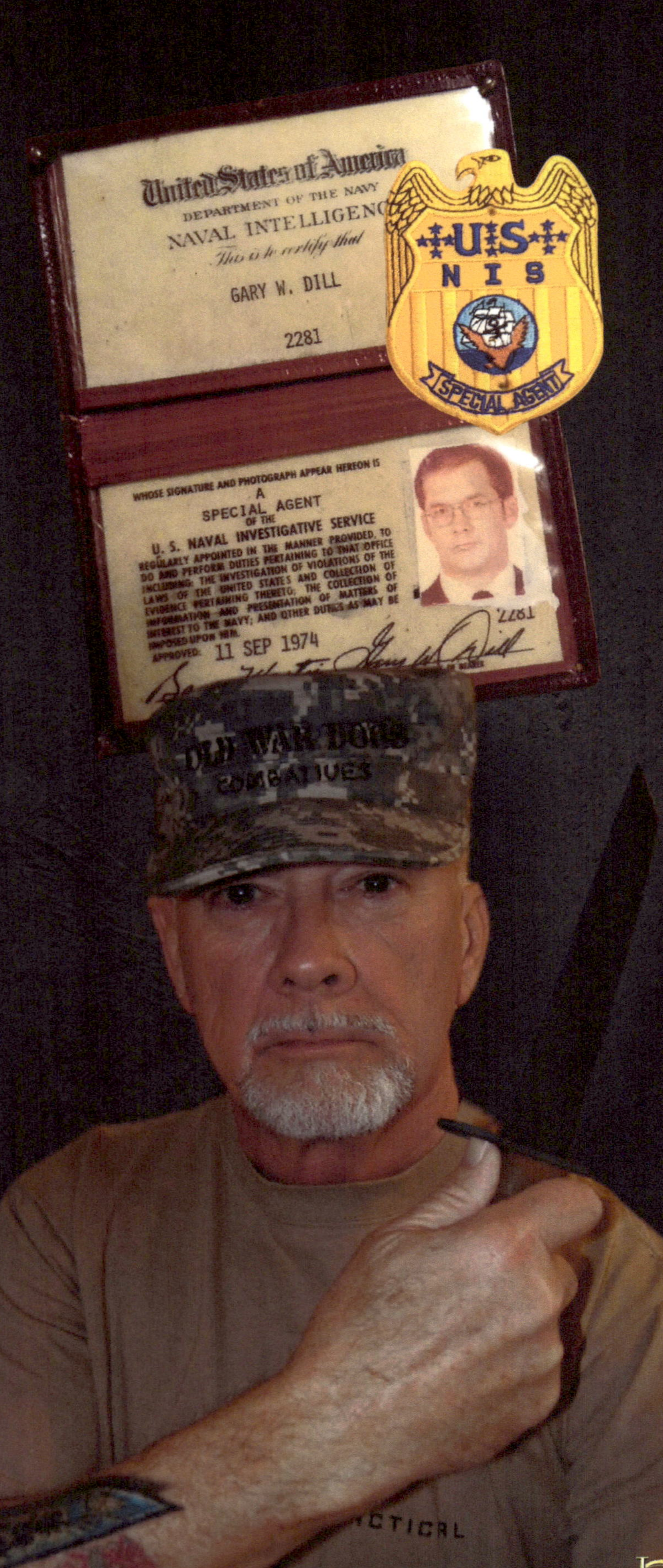

As part of my JKD knife combat training, I emphasize developing the mindset of terminating or seriously disabling the enemy. James Lee would lecture our small JKD class, stating, "If you want to be a real JKD fighter, you must develop the Killer Instinct."

Still on active military duty at this time, having just returned from Vietnam, I understood exactly what he meant.

The combatant must be willing and able to take out the enemy without hesitation, without remorse. It is a matter of survival with attitude. You have to work this out in your own mind, your own moral compass, as to what you are willing to do in order to survive.

Waiting until the fight starts to cope with this philosophical issue is too late. If you do, you will be distracted, and you will be dead.

Hesitation kills. You must already resolve it within yourself so that when the moment arises when you are facing your enemy, you will not hesitate to attack and defend yourself. When you attack with your knife, it should be done immediately in the blink of an eye.

You need to reflect the mindset of the Samurai and terminate your opponent without hesitation or compassion. The only thing on your mind should be the elimination of the threat of your enemy. Do not think about what he can do to you, but what you will do to him.

My personal JKD combat knife system demonstrates an arsenal of effective and devastating blade techniques based upon the original Oakland JKD techniques and tactics, along with some "specialized" techniques acquired during my military and intelligence career.

We use only two combat grips, the SABRE GRIP and the REVERSE GRIP.

Let's make it clear: on the battlefield or on the street, you are not dueling with a knife. There should be no fancy moves like in the movies. You use the knife to terminate or seriously wound the enemy during combat when a firearm is not accessible.

There is no "fairness" in battle; you either win or lose. You fight to survive with whatever means are available. The knife is used as your backup weapon. Or you may be involved on a mission where you must use stealth and silence, and the knife or empty-hand techniques are the only tools you can use.

While in the military and law enforcement, I always carried a backup knife, which was my ace up my sleeve. You can dispatch the enemy efficiently and quickly if you are properly trained with a knife. But the keywords here are "properly trained."

You have to know how to grip the knife, how to position your hands, how to utilize the appropriate stance, how to recognize the best and most accessible target, and most importantly, how to execute the most appropriate and efficient knife techniques during your attack.

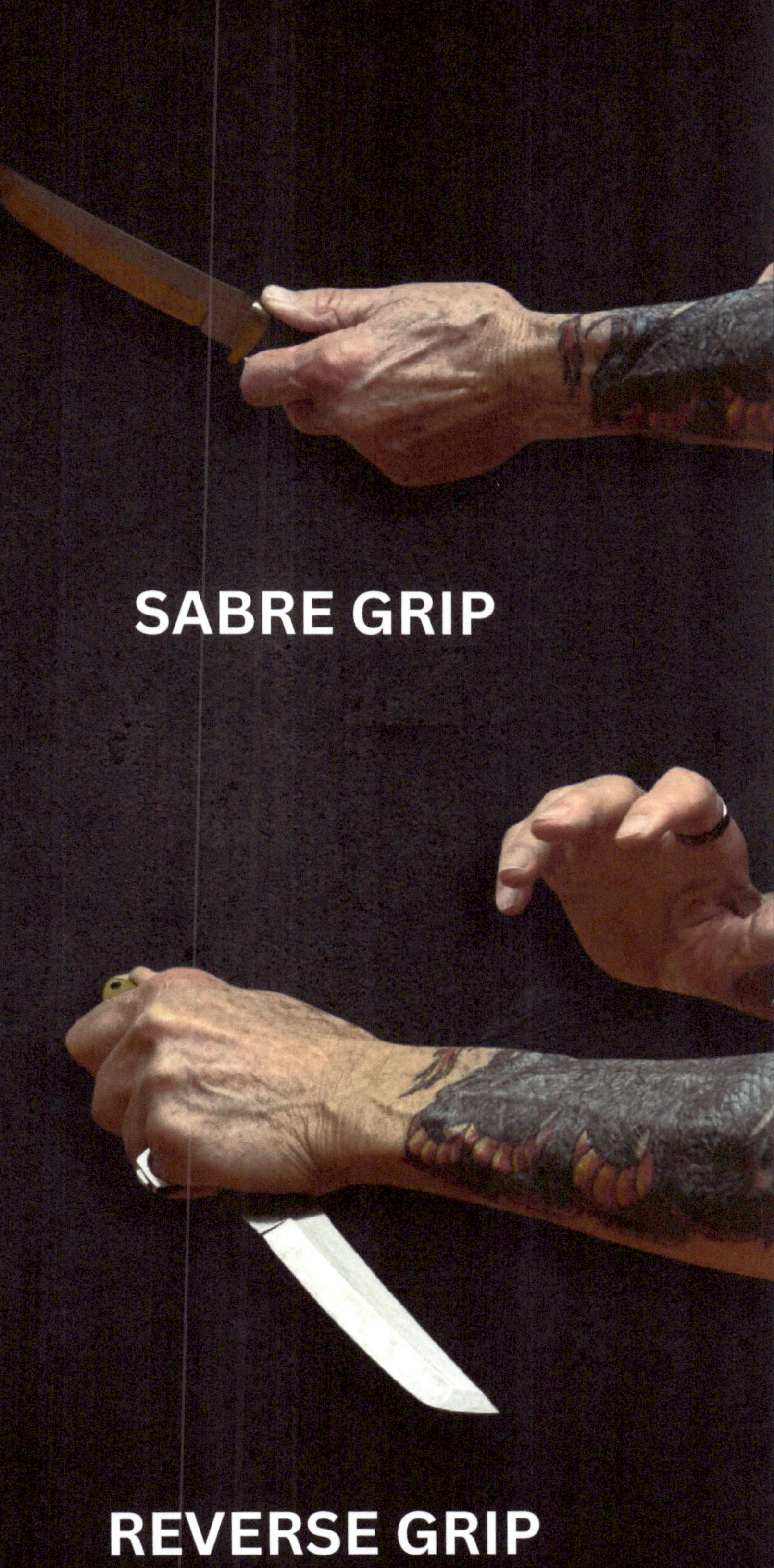

This is where Jeet Kune Do comes into the picture.

From my own real-life combat experience, I believe that the original JKD is one of the world's most effective combat martial arts today.

JKD is simple, direct, and deceptive. There is no sport, rituals, aesthetics, or competition in JKD. It is reality-based combat. When trained in the original JKD and put a knife in your hand, you now have a deadly and efficient knife-fighting system.

DILL'S PRINCIPLES OF JKD KNIFE FIGHTING

Only use a knife when your life is at stake or serious bodily injury. No exceptions

In my system, we use only two grips: Sabre or Reverse. They both have their own dynamics and purposes.

Use a few knife techniques that work best for you. Train with them, get them down to a pure conditioned reflex. Be able to apply them without thinking. Thinking is your enemy in combat; when fighting you must rely on "muscle memory."

Attack and cut whatever part of his body is closest to you. For example, when the opponent is facing you in a stance, cut his hand closest to you. Hack away and eliminate his ability to block your knife strikes. Also, psychological shock will set in

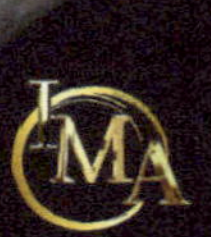

and make it easier to stop the enemy's threat.

Draw first blood and induce psychological shock. Most people have not been in actual combat and have not experienced serious bleeding. Upon realizing that they have been cut and are bleeding, when in combat many will go into psychological shock, and realize that their life is now in serious danger.

Psychological shock is the knife fighter's best tool because it can neutralize the enemy quicker than the actual wound.

Attack with resolve and without hesitation. When in actual combat, practical training and conditioned reflexes must take over. Long before he goes into combat, one must work out any moral issues they may have regarding injuring or taking the life of an enemy.

The battlefield is not the time or place to wrestle with this issue. In combat, there is no time for hesitation; you must take action immediately............before your enemy does.

Maintain forward energy. Be aggressive! Real combat is not the place to be passive or defensive. Defensive tactics result in giving your opponent more opportunity to terminate you. To survive combat, you must be aggressive, keep pressing in on your opponent, and do not give him any time to respond or counterattack.

Do not try to intimidate with the knife. The purpose of the knife on the battlefield is to terminate the enemy.

Combat is not the time to "play" with an enemy, or to try to scare him. Just move in accordingly and take him out without hesitation. Real street combat is not like the make-believe movie fighting. You need to finish the knife combat within a few seconds. The longer you fight, the more chances he has to injure or kill you.

Be quick, if you are slow in combat you probably won't survive. Regardless of how many knife techniques you may know, if they don't get to the target, they are worthless. Speed is everything. As well as learning effective knife tactics, you must also train in executing them quickly.

Train, train, train.

Keep your movements minimal, simple, and direct. Forget what you see in the movies. All of those fancy moves are not functional in real knife combat. Keep your attack simple and direct, no dojo ballerina moves.

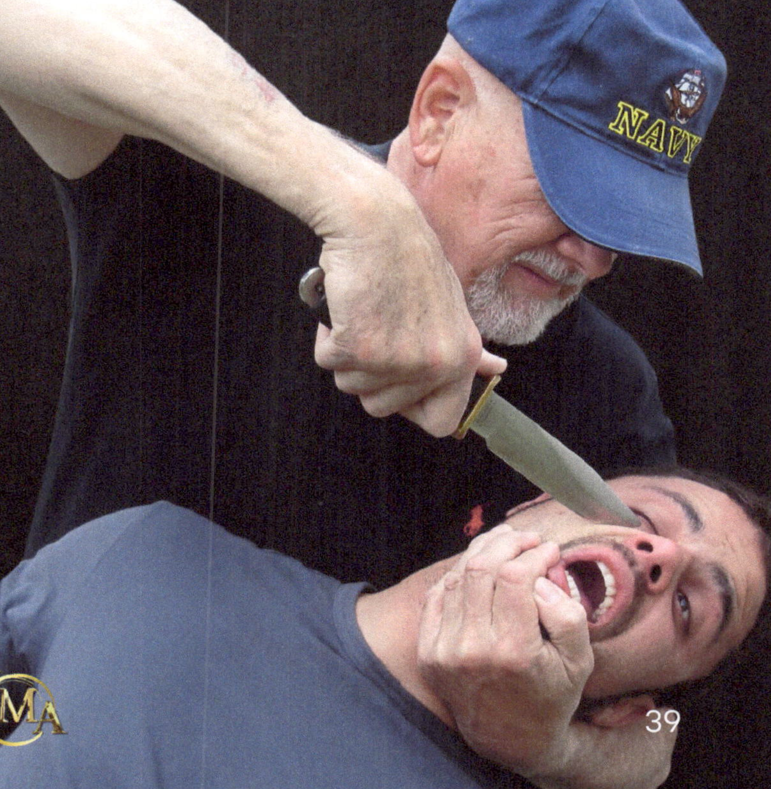

The fewer moves you execute in knife combat, the fewer openings you give your opponent, and the fewer opportunities for his counterattack.

Use footwork for evasion and attack. JKD footwork works great for knife applications because of the emphasis on angular movements and the forward lunge with a straight knife thrust. (Bruce Lee incorporated this move from fencing.)

Maintain your centerline when positioning your knife. Just as in JKD, the knife combatant needs to protect his vital organs and utilize the closed centerline theory from Wing Chun. As in JKD, lead with your strongest and most coordinated hand, thus the knife should be in the leading hand.

he knife is there to protect you, not you protecting the knife. If the opponent wants to get to you, he must be able to try to get through your knife, which will end poorly for him.

Be familiar with critical targets on your opponent. Attack to terminate or seriously disable. Attack specific targets such as the throat, side of the neck, solar plexus, groin, the eye, supra sternal notch, subclavian region, base of the skull, and kidney. Become very familiar with these target areas.

These knife-fighting principles can be very devastating when applied using the original JKD techniques and in conjunction with proper mental and psychological preparation.

About the Author

Professor Gary Dill has been active in JKD for 53 years and is one of the few original students still living (1971 – Present.) Dill trained in JKD at the Oakland school under James Lee with Bruce Lee being the head instructor. He is the founder and Chief Instructor of the Jeet Kune Do Association (founded in 1991.) Dill spent many years in the military (Vietnam veteran, Special Agent with NCIS (Office of Naval Intelligence), and was a state criminal investigator working narcotics, homicides, organized crime, and police corruption.

While a Special Agent with NCIS, Dill was a close-quarters combat (CQC) and firearms instructor. Also, he was the senior police defensive tactics instructor for the state of Oklahoma police certification agency (CLEET.) He worked as a private military "contractor" and taught CQC and knife tactics to military spec ops and Homeland Security personnel.

Professor Gary Dill is a regular contributor to IMA Magazine. Catch his monthly column and insight in every issue.

He can be contacted at pdilljkd@aol.com , and his website is www.jkd-garydill.com .

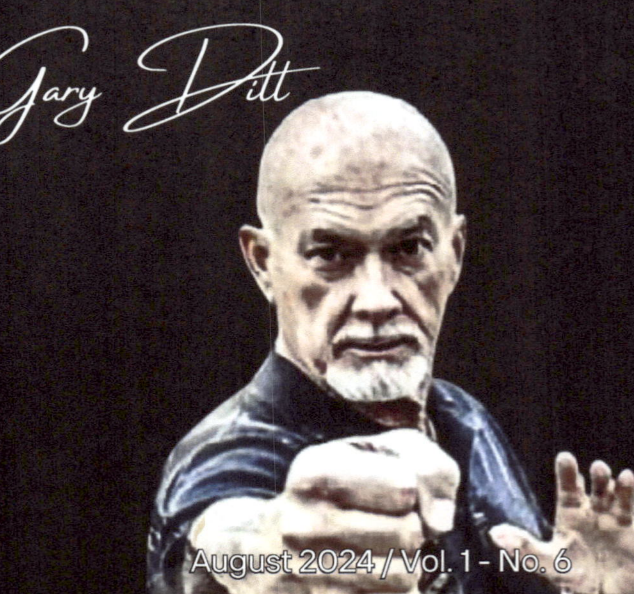

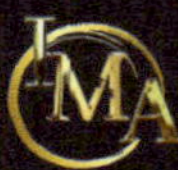

SANDOKAN

THE CUTTING EDGE MARTIAL ART

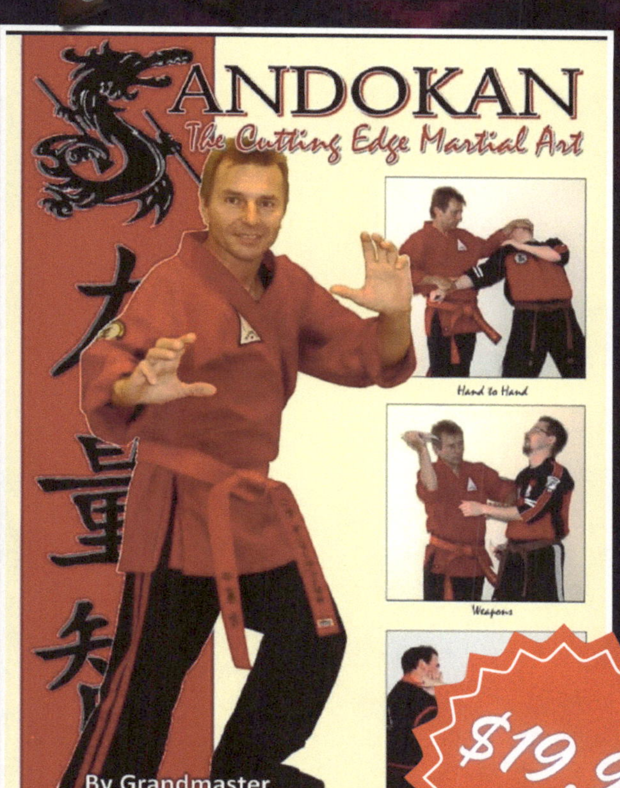

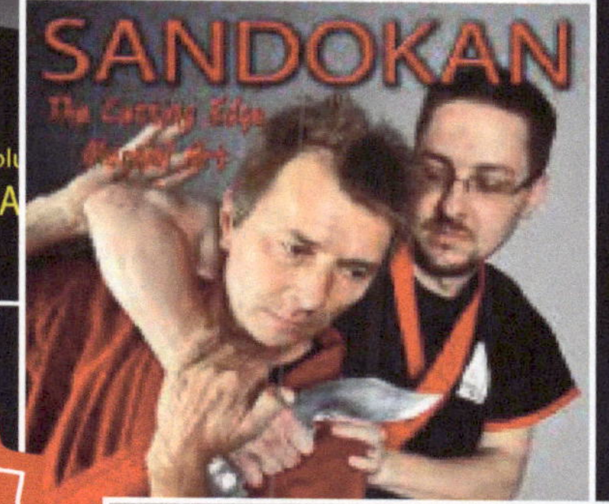

Basic Street Knife Defense DVD 1

$19.95

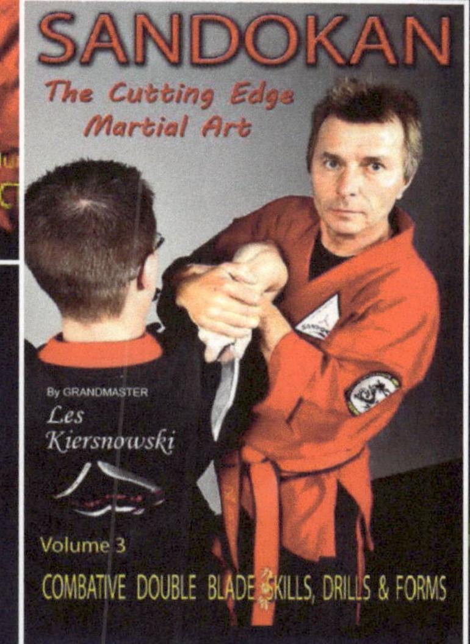

Tactical Knife Disarms & Control DVD 2

$19.95

Combative Double Blade Drills & Forms DVD 3

$19.95

The Sandokan system is based on physics, principles of martial science, and the science of anatomy. Achieving this martial arts system has encompassed many years of research and practical development. It is a system based on the perfecting of body positioning for maximum output of energy.

293 pages English   2019 7 x 0.66 x 10 inch

ORDER NOW

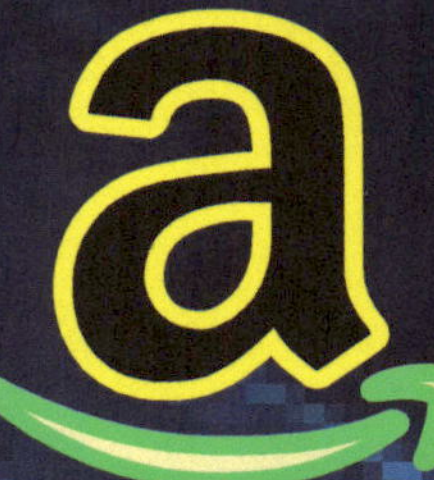

lechkiersnowski@gmail.com
AVAILABLE ON AMAZON.COM

AVAILABLE NOW

WING CHUN KUNG FU

Rules of Engagement

By Clark Tang

Wing Chun Kung Fu, with roots embedded deeply in Chinese martial arts, is a martial art focused on practical self-defense, efficiency, and the enhancement of the human spirit.

One of the modern torchbearers of this art is Sifu Clark Tang, an esteemed practitioner and teacher whose journey spans almost 50 years. Sifu Tang's interpretation of Wing Chun goes beyond physical prowess. it immerses one in a philosophical approach that integrates mind, body, and spirit.

As a martial artist, one must hold to the true values of the way of the warriors. Majority of people don't know martial arts, only a few among these individuals, may know and very effective of using martial arts.

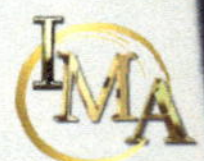

However, one must know that great power comes with great responsibilities. One should never use your martial arts for anything else except for honor, defending yourself and loved ones, and preserving the art. The bottom line is that martial arts is using for the good.

At the heart of his teachings are the "Fighting Rules of Engagement ", designed to guide practitioners not only in combat but also in life.

These following rules can be applied in almost any given situation.

Talk-Fu

The first principle, Talk-Fu, emphasizes the power of communication. If tension arises, it advises one to diffuse the situation through dialogue first.

In Tang's words,

"The worst situations should be resolved peacefully with good mannerism, sincere attitude, and good faith."

This approach reflects a profound understanding of human nature and underscores the importance of seeking peaceful resolutions whenever possible.

Walk-Fu

If talking fails, Sifu Tang introduces Walk-Fu.

In this principle, one is encouraged to remove themselves from the situation if the other party remains irrational or aggressive. Sometimes Talk-Fu may not work due to many reasons or circumstances such as talking to idiots or ignorant individuals who don't deserve your attention at all, he explains.

"Walking away is not a sign of Cowardice but a testament to one's wisdom and control."

Kung-Fu

When peaceful measures prove futile, and if one is left with no other option, only then do they resort to Kung-Fu, the physical execution of Wing Chun techniques.

"It is only to be used as a last resort,"

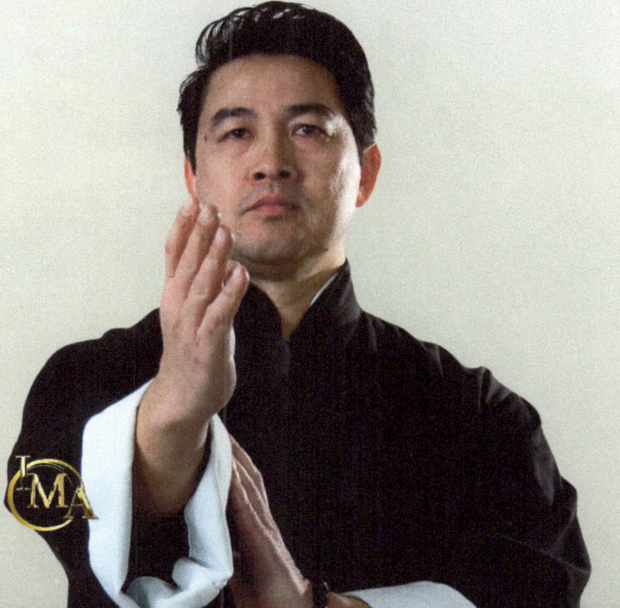

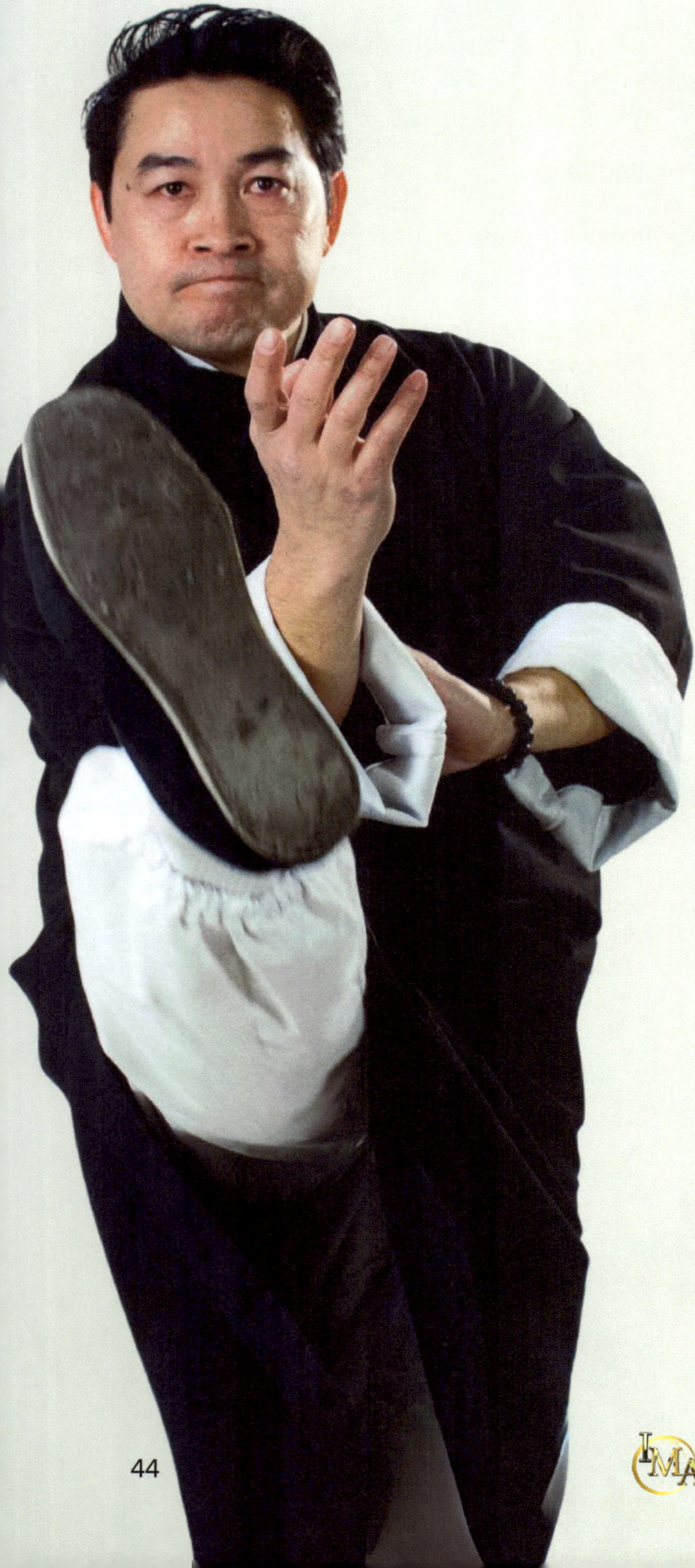

Gun-Fu

In Sifu Tang's perspective, one must adapt to the changing times.

He introduces Gun-Fu, acknowledging the sobering reality that sometimes, traditional martial arts are not enough.

In life-threatening situations involving deadly weapons, he believes that proper, responsible use of firearms can be necessary.

He advises,

"Please consult your firearms coach and do your own research with deep understanding and treat it with love and respect of its law."

A Philosophy for Life Sifu Clark Tang's life embodies the martial philosophy of Wing Chun.

He continuously adapts and refines his knowledge, seeking to improve himself physically, mentally, and spiritually. His teachings transcend combat; they aspire to shape better fathers, husbands, friends, and ultimately, better human beings.

These are the true marks of a martial artist, cultivated not just through mastery of techniques but through a harmonious balance of mind, body, and spirit.

Sifu Tang's Wing Chun is not just about fighting; it's about living. It's about carrying the virtues of respect, humility, and love into every aspect of life.

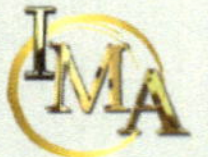

As he fittingly puts it, the ultimate goal in Wing Chun and in life is to embody Love, Peace, and Compassion.

As a martial artist, one must hold to the true values of the way of the warriors. Majority of people don't know martial arts, only a few among these individuals, may know and very effective of using martial arts. However, one must know that great power comes with great responsibilities.

Never use your martial arts for anything else except for honor, defending yourself and loved ones, and preserving the art.

The bottom line is that martial arts is using for the good. After many years in the martial arts world and community, which is almost 50 years journey, Sifu Tang came up with The Fighting Rules of Engagement.

As a lifelong martial art practitioner with various systems and styles of martial arts, he came to love Wing Chun Kung Fu and the journey didn't stop there.

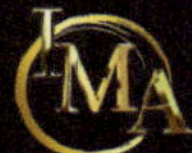

Wing Chun Kung Fu is all about adapting and refining of what we learn and make it better and better as we age gracefully and happily.

Sifu Clark Tang always seeking ways to improve myself physically, mentally and spiritually under the principles of Wing Chun Kung Fu under God's love and grace.

If you're a father, how can you be the best father as you can be. If you're a husband, how can you be the best husband as you can be. If you are a friend, how can you be the best friend that you can be.

All in all, the ultimate goal of life is Love, Peace, Compassion, Unity and Harmony. I love you all.

Clark Tang

About the Author

Sifu Clark started interest in Martial Arts at the 4. His quest for an understanding of Martial Arts was an everlasting.

Inspired by Master Ti Lung and later by Master Bruce Lee, Wing Chun Gung Fu was always his goal to study. But there was not any Wing Chun Gung Fu school around him at the time, so he started to study American Kenpo Karate and Kickboxing with Sensei Paul Hock's school.

Later he met Sensei Thomas Martin, and I asked a permission from Sensei Paul Hock to study under Sensei Thomas Martin. Later he trained with Thomas Martin.

He continued to learn various other arts like Tae Kwon Do, Tai Chi and other martial arts styles. But his heart was always drawn to Wing Chun Gung Fu.

Clark later became CEO and founder of the Wing Chun Temple in Orange County California. Developing young minds in the art of Wing Chun.

The vision of his legacy has history are being passed onto others through his teachings and his school.

WING CHUN TEMPLE School's Mission and Vision: WING CHUN TEMPLE is not just another martial arts school, nor just another Wing Chun Kwoon; it's an ALL- inclusive Martial Arts School by combining the old way of learning into the modern world that we're living in.

For more information contact Sifu Clark Tang www.WingChunTemple.com

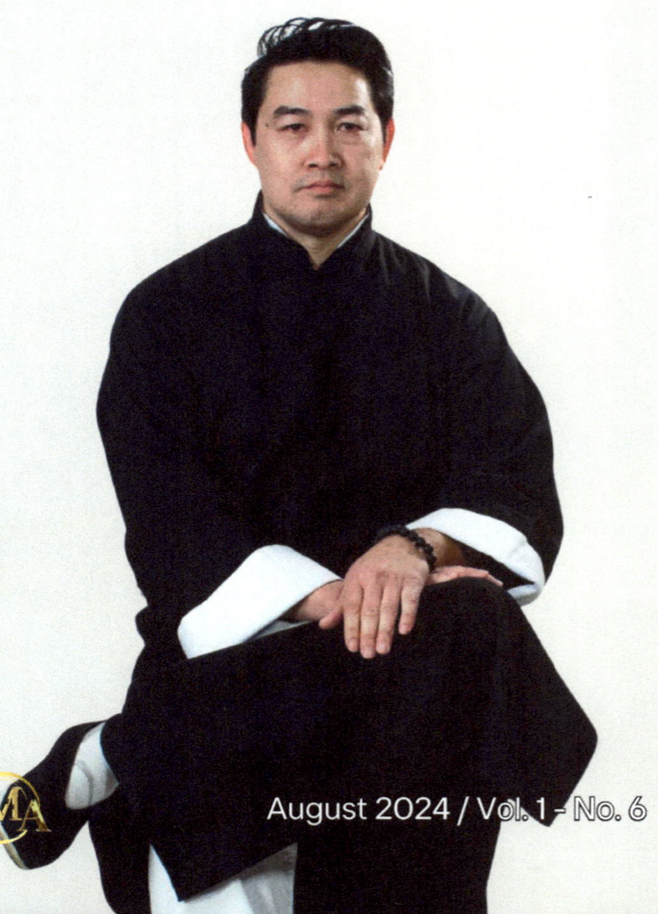

KENPO KARATE 2024 HALL OF FAME

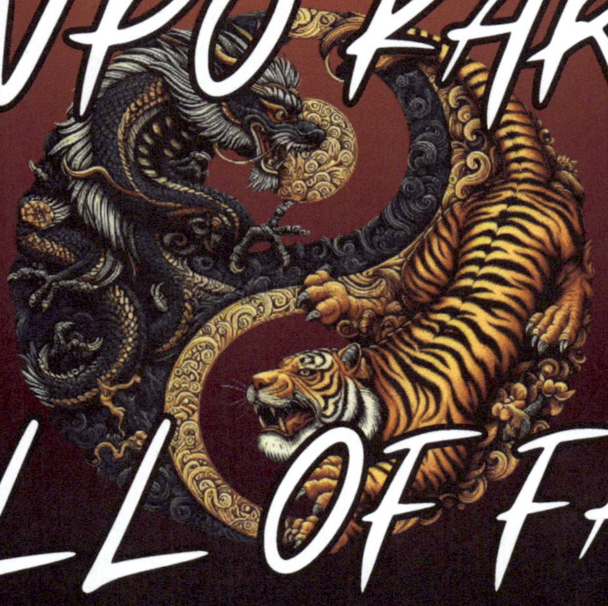

By Allen Woodman Photography by Allen Woodman / Dan Kennedy / Sally Steele

The 2024 KENPO Karate Hall of Fame (KKHOF) event, hosted by Master Paul Casey, took place this past June at the beautiful downtown California Hotel and Casino in Las Vegas. The event, celebrated from June 14-15, brought together the crème de la crème of the martial arts world.

The ceremony started with a vibrant traditional Hawaiian hula performance by Kuma Lua Michelle Manu, recently featured on the cover of International Martial Arts Magazine. This was followed by short speeches and introductions, setting the stage for prominent instructors' informative and elective seminars.

The event dove into action-packed seminars led by elite Kenpo instructors from around the globe.

The event saw special performances and presentations including the KKHOF demonstrations featuring guests like Marty Zaninovich, Steve Rodarte, and Todd Durgan covering a spectrum of techniques from fundamental maneuvers to advanced knife fighting.

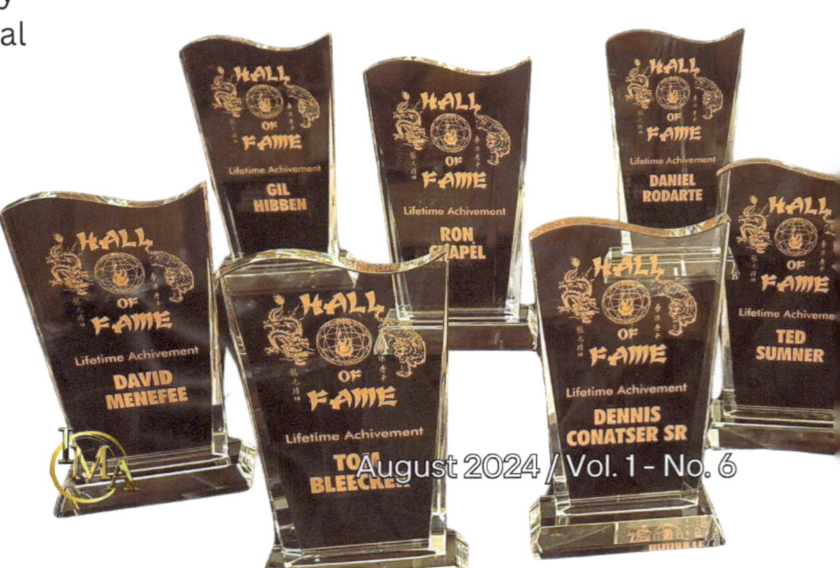

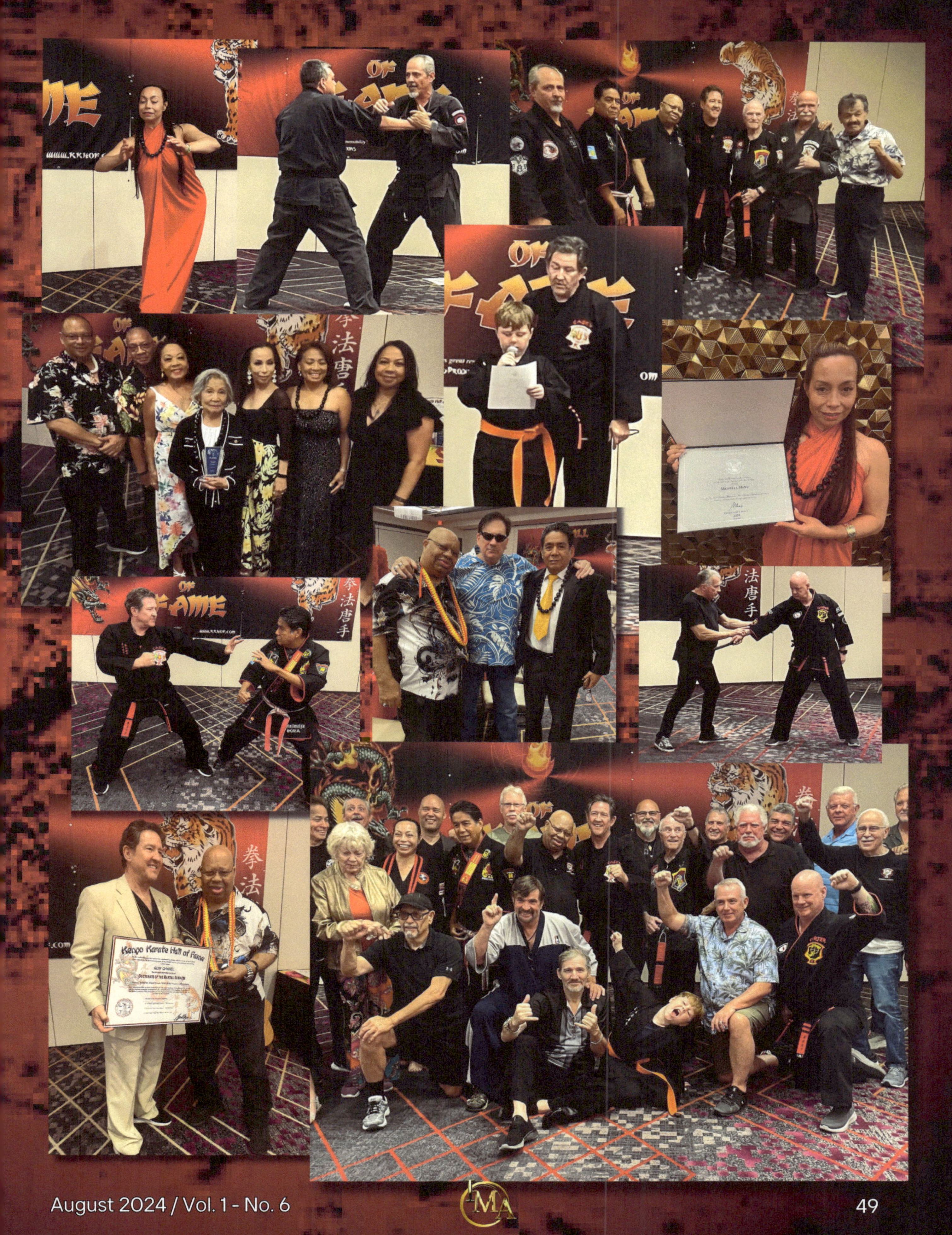

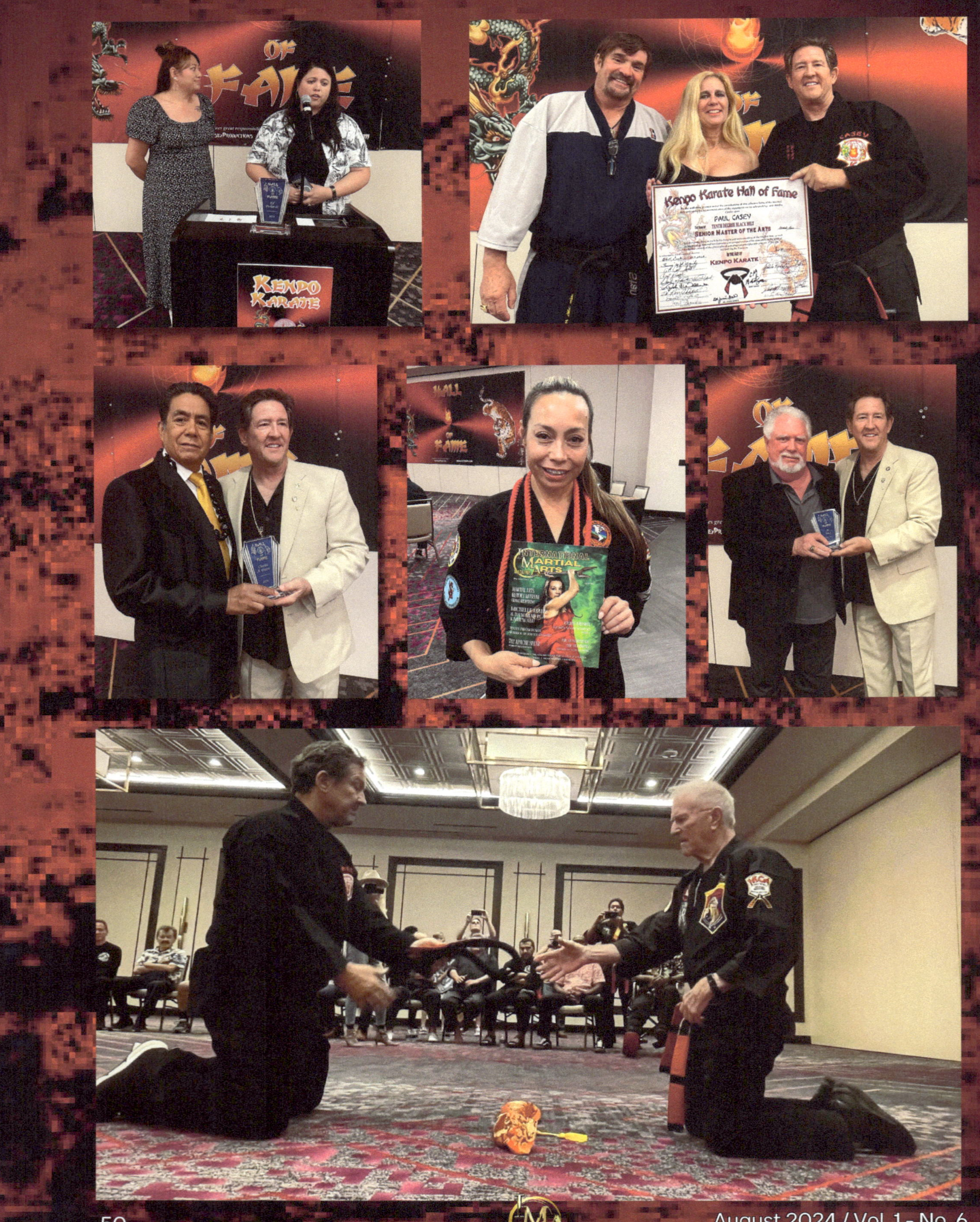

The event truly lived up to its theme with numerous highlights, including Lifetime Achievement Awards, KKHOF inductions, seminars, a Hawaiian Luau, entertainment, and more.

KKHOF, known for honoring the greatest martial artists from over fourteen styles, systems, and disciplines, celebrated the following awards:

Lifetime Achievement Awards

- Dennis Conatser, Sr
- Daniel Rodarte
- Ted Sumner
- Gil Hibben
- David Menefee
- Tom Bleecker
- Ron Chapél

Golden Dragon Award

- Todd Durgan

The highlight of a heartfelt ceremony was Paul Casey's promotion to 10th-degree black belt, officiated by Kenpo legend Chuck Sullivan, a direct student of Ed Parker Sr.

Family members occasionally accepted awards on behalf of recipients who could not be present, such as the daughters of Ed Parker Jr. and George Lazenby.

The celebration continued with the Saturday Awards Ceremony Hawaiian Luau, special presentations, inductions, displays, and a red-carpet photo opportunity.

Among the notable attendees were martial arts ICON Frank Dux and International Martial Arts Magazine editor and publisher Allen Woodman as well as Tournament promoter Stan Witz.

2024 KKHOF Inductees

- Kailani Koa
- Charles A. Dixon
- Ralph Castro
- Rob Castro
- Michelle Manu
- David German
- Fred Villari
- Ed Parker II
- Al Tracy
- David Crouch
- Patrick Strong
- Lorenzo Jimenez
- David Lee Roth
- George Lazenby

The 2024 KKHOF event was a fantastic weekend of information sharing, community bonding, and delicious food, making it a memorable affair for all guests.

For More Information
Website: [https://kkhof.com]

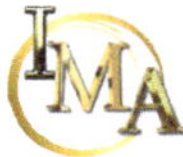

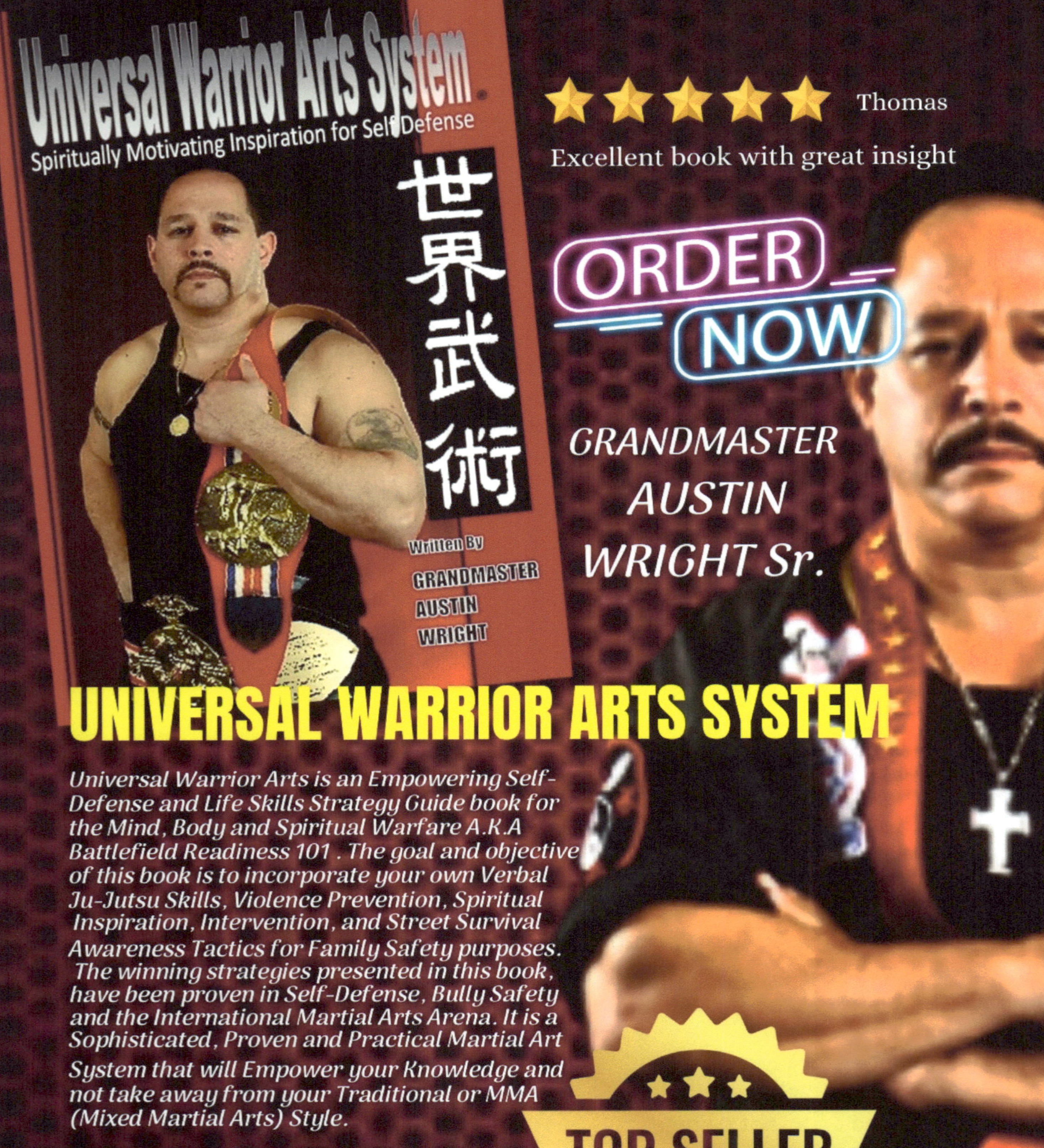

Universal Warrior Arts System
Spiritually Motivating Inspiration for Self Defense
世界武術
Written By
GRANDMASTER
AUSTIN
WRIGHT
Thomas
Excellent book with great insight
ORDER
NOW
GRANDMASTER
AUSTIN
WRIGHT Sr.
UNIVERSAL WARRIOR ARTS SYSTEM
Universal Warrior Arts is an Empowering Self-Defense and Life Skills Strategy Guide book for the Mind, Body and Spiritual Warfare A.K.A Battlefield Readiness 101 . The goal and objective of this book is to incorporate your own Verbal Ju-Jutsu Skills, Violence Prevention, Spiritual Inspiration, Intervention, and Street Survival Awareness Tactics for Family Safety purposes. The winning strategies presented in this book, have been proven in Self-Defense, Bully Safety and the International Martial Arts Arena. It is a Sophisticated, Proven and Practical Martial Art System that will Empower your Knowledge and not take away from your Traditional or MMA (Mixed Martial Arts) Style.
Language : English
Paperback : 182 pages
Dimensions : 7 x 0.71 x 10 inches
TOP SELLER
AVAILABLE ON AMAZON.COM

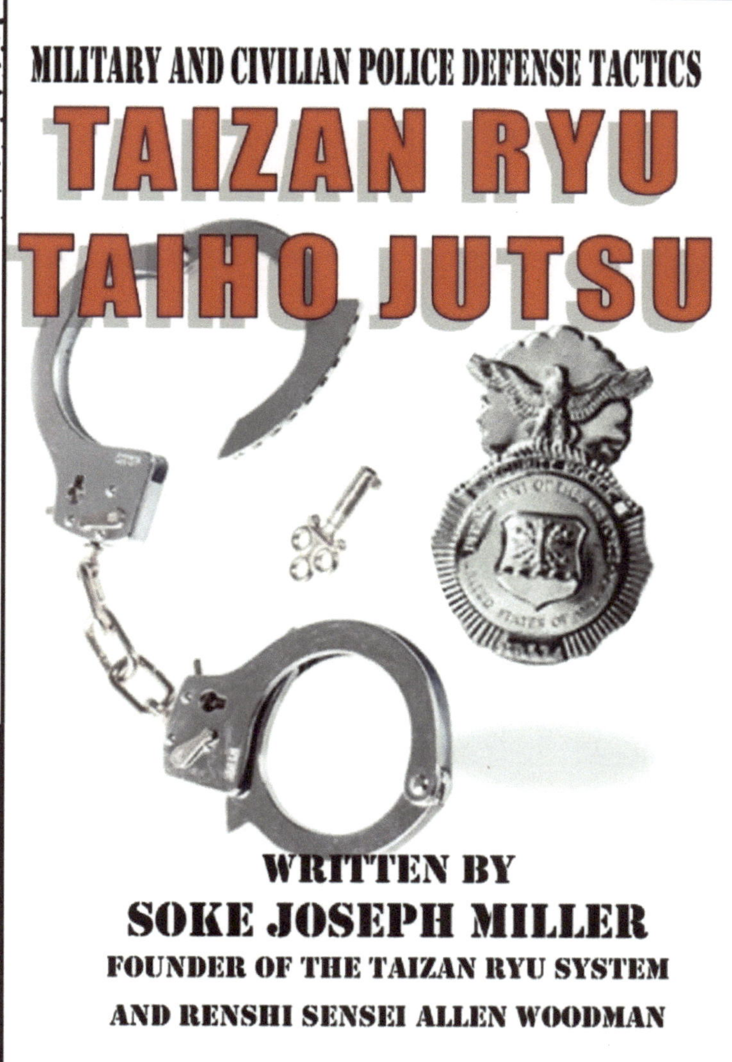

ORDER NOW

$9.95

BOOK &DVD

SOLD SEPERATLY

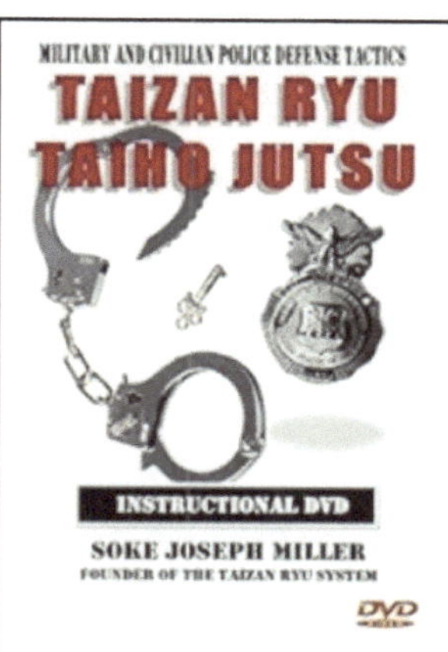

90 pages
English
Publication date
February 7, 2011
6 x 0.21 x 9 inches

POLICE APPREHENSION & SELF-DEFENSE PROGRAM

Taizan Ryu Taiho Jutsu founded by Soke Joe Miller, a 50 year veteran of martial arts, 9th degree black belt and the leading authority and founder of Taizan Ryu Taiho Jutsu system. This complete manual has all 18 techniques that have been patented by the U.S. Government to train both Civilian and military police in correct apprehension and arrest procedures and techniques that are both effective and useful in the field.

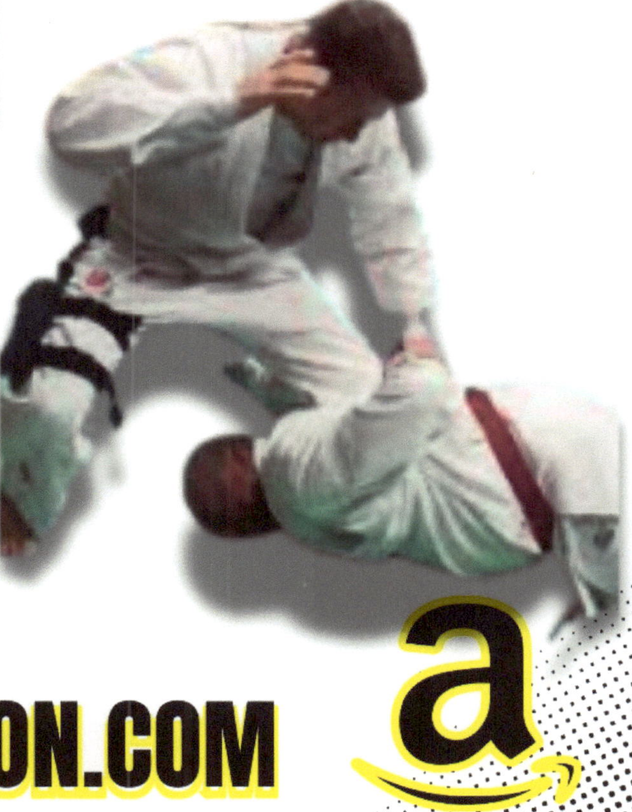

PLUS a instructional DVD available now!

AVAILABLE ON AMAZON.COM

THE HEALING TOUCH

MONTHLY COLUMN By Joe Miller

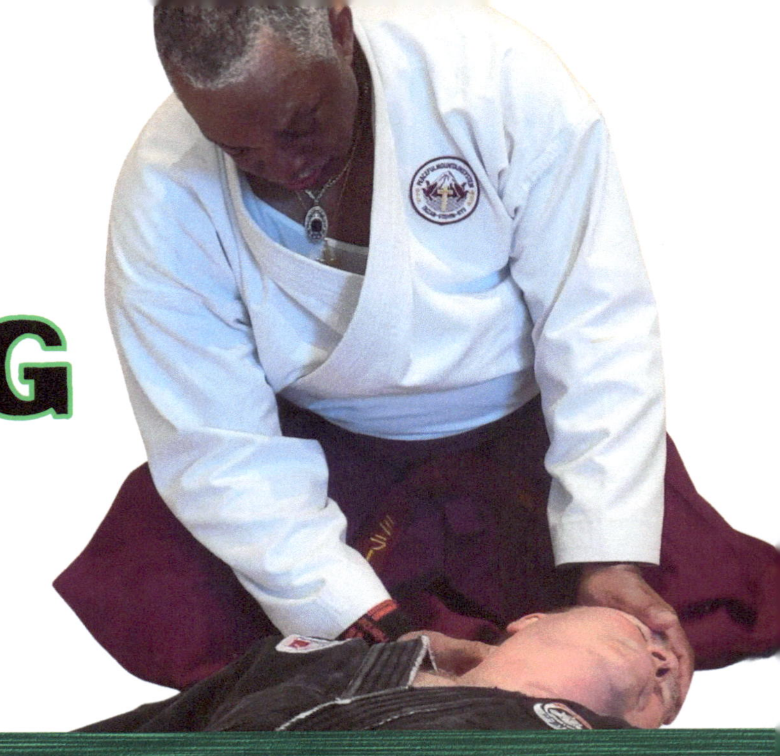

The Pericardium Meridian

The Pericardium Meridian, also known as the Heart Protector Meridian, follows a specific pathway on the body:

Its Starting Point begins in the center of the chest, around the pericardium.

The Pathway travels outward along the chest, through the armpit, and down the inner side of the arm. It runs between the biceps and triceps muscles, through the elbow crease, down the forearm, and through the center of the wrist.

The Ending Point terminates at the tip of the middle finger.

There are many Tsubo points on the Pericardium Meridian.

Its Functions:

The Pericardium Meridian has several important functions:

Protection: It acts as a protective layer for the heart, both physically and energetically, safeguarding it from external pathogenic factors.

Regulation of Emotions is closely associated with the mind and emotions, especially those related to joy, love, and sadness.

The Circulation of Qi and Blood helps regulate the flow of KI (vital energy) and blood in the body, ensuring that the heart functions efficiently.

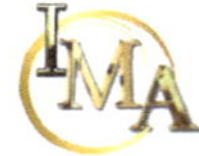

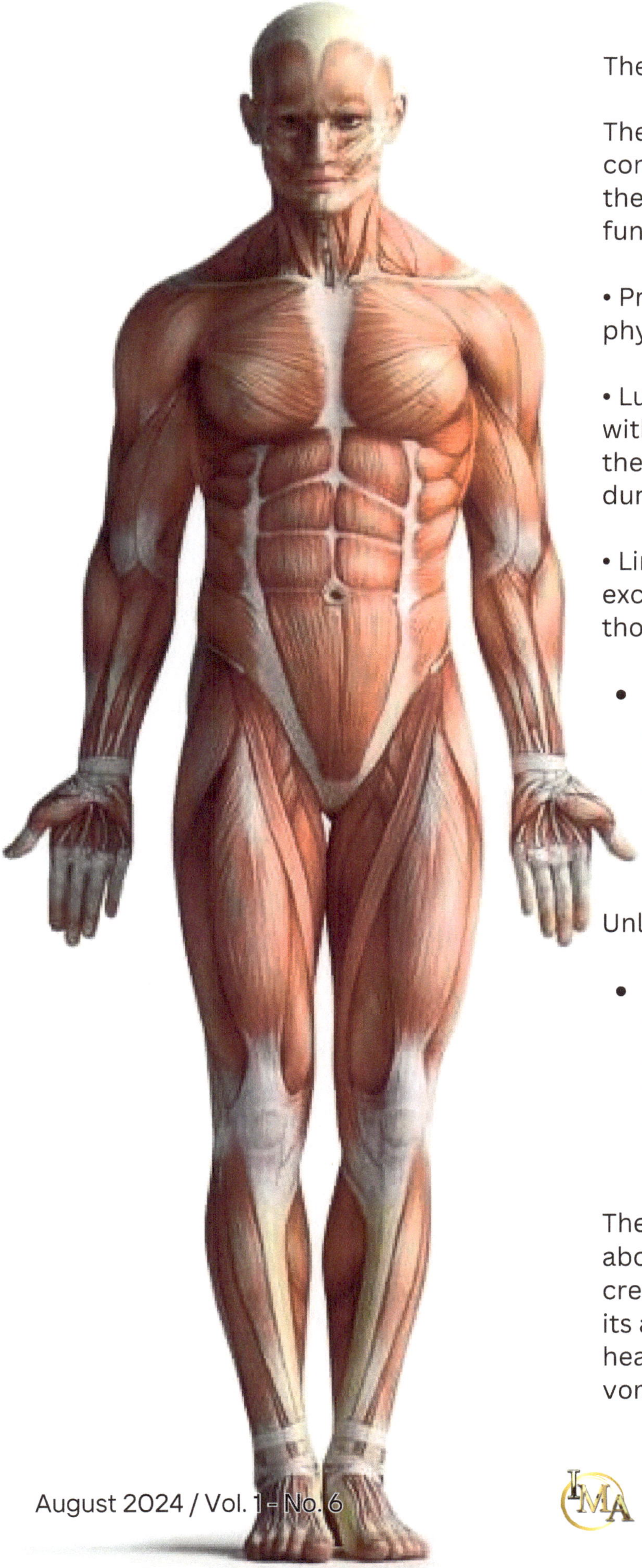

The Pericardium Organ 1. Physical Role:

The pericardium is a double-walled sac containing the heart and the roots of the major blood vessels. Its primary functions are:

• Protection protects the heart from physical trauma and infections.

• Lubrication: The pericardial fluid within the sac reduces friction between the heart and surrounding structures during heartbeats.

• Limits Heart Motion: It restricts excessive heart movement within the thorax.

• Energetic Role in TCM: In TJM, the pericardium is viewed not just as a physical structure but as a vital energy center that influences emotional health, heart health, and overall vitality.

Unlocking of the Pericardium Meridian

• Shiatsu application to this Meridian line will Stimulate specific points along the Pericardium Meridian, which can have various therapeutic effects. Some key points include: Therapeutic Potential

The Pericardium Meridian is Located about two inches above the wrist crease on the inner arm; it is known for its ability to calm the mind, regulate the heart, and alleviate nausea and vomiting.

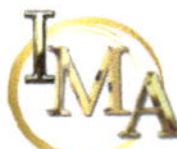

Shiatsu application to the pericardium meridian is used to clear heat from the heart and calm the spirit.

- Effects on the Heart Muscle: Stimulating the Pericardium Meridian can influence the heart muscle in several ways:

• Regulation of Heart Rate: Balancing the flow of KI and blood can help normalize the heart rate.

• Stress Reduction: By calming the mind and alleviating emotional stress, it can reduce the physical strain on the heart.

• Improvement of Circulation: Enhanced blood flow can improve the nourishment and oxygenation of the heart muscle, supporting its overall health and function.

In conclusion the Pericardium Meridian plays a crucial role in protecting and supporting heart health, both physically and energetically.

Its regulation of emotions and promotion of smooth KI and blood flow contribute to overall well-being.

Understanding and utilizing this meridian in practices such as acupuncture and Shiatsu can provide significant health benefits, particularly for the cardiovascular system and emotional health.

About the Author

Soke Joseph Miller has been involved for more than six decades. Spending many of his formative years in Japan mastering the art of Hakko-Ryu Jujitsu under its founder Okuyama sensei.

Along with his traditional martial arts training, he also underwent years of hands-on training and study of Japanese Shiatsu (Acupressure).

After many years of practice, he was given a license to practice the art of healing and has been doing so for many years. His personal belief is that God has given him the ability to help heal the human body, and his teachers gave him the understanding of how to do it.

Soke Joe Miller has also Co-Authored the book The Healing Touch Complete with Allen Woodman. Soke Joe Miller teaches in his own school in Hachioji, Japan as well as conducts international seminars upon request.

For more information please feel free to contact Joe miller via facebook @ Soke Joseph Miller or through his website ww.peacefulmountainsystemtaizanryu. site

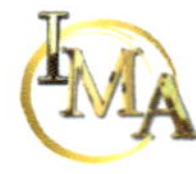

★★★★★ Tony B.

That's a really good book. Picture, text, Everything is so detailed

★★★★★ Kennete Kleese

The book is understandable whether you are a beginner or advance student or professional of any style of massage

★★★★★ Barry Southam

Great text to add to your library.

Learn the ancient art of shiatsu massage and its healing abilities.Relieve stress and aches while healing the body naturally through the Japanese art of acute finger pressure through this insightful and useful guide. With full-color photos and artwork of the human anatomy and step by step practice guides to instruct you from student to fully certified practitioner. In Japan, the practice of finger pressure massage known as Shiatsu is a highly respected, professional skill that uses the meridians and blood flow to naturally heal the body. Shiatsu can reduce tension and even alleviate health issues. Includes Test out portions of the text to gain full credentials in this amazing healing method from Asia.

LIMITED

$69.95

FREE DELIVERY

- Language : English
- Paperback : 299 pages
- Dimensions : 7 x 0.71 x 10 inches

QUALITY GUARANTEED

AVAILABLE ON AMAZON.COM

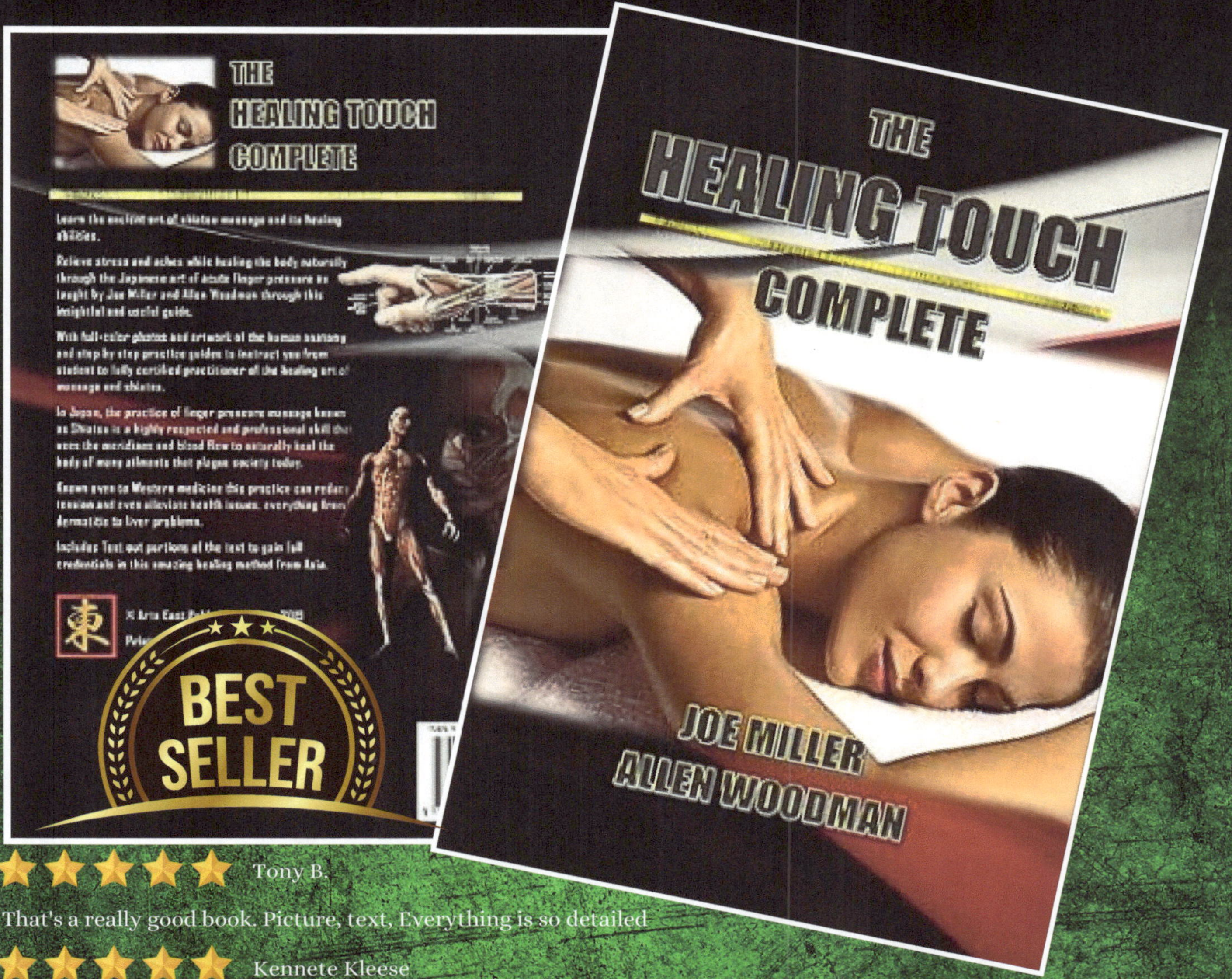

www.ingramcontent.com/pod-product-compliance
Lightning Source LLC
Chambersburg PA
CBHW040136240726
48664CB00002B/502